American Psychiatry and Homosexuality
An Oral History

HARRINGTON PARK PRESS®
Titles of Related Interest

Handbook of LGBT Issues in Community Mental Health edited by Ronald E. Hellman and Jack Drescher

Lesbian and Bisexual Women's Mental Health edited by Robin M. Mathy and Shelly K. Kerr

Lesbians, Feminism, and Psychoanalysis: The Second Wave edited by Judith M. Glassgold and Suzanne Iasenza

Relationship Therapy with Same-Sex Couples edited by Jerry J. Bigner and Joseph Wetchler

Anything But Straight: Unmasking the Scandals and Lies Behind the Ex-Gay Myth by Wayne R. Besen

Psychotherapy with Gay Men and Lesbians: Contemporary Dynamic Approaches by Jack Drescher, Ann D'Ercole, and Erica Schoenberg

The Mental Health Professions and Homosexuality: International Perspectives edited by Vittorio Lingiardi and Jack Drescher

The Therapist's Notebook for Lesbian, Gay, and Bisexual Clients: Homework, Handouts, and Activities for Use in Psychotherapy edited by Joy S. Whitman and Cynthia J. Boyd

Sex, Cells, and Same-Sex Desire: The Biology of Sexual Preference edited by John P. De Cecco and David Allen Parker

Gay and Lesbian Mental Health: A Sourcebook for Practitioners edited by Christopher J. Alexander

American Psychiatry and Homosexuality
An Oral History

Jack Drescher, MD
Joseph P. Merlino, MD, MPA
Editors

Routledge
Taylor & Francis Group
LONDON AND NEW YORK

First published by

Harrington Park Press®, the trade division of The Haworth Press, Inc., 10 Alice Street, Binghamton, NY 13904-1580.

Published 2016 by
Routledge
711 Third Avenue, New York, NY 10017

and by Routledge
2 Park Square, Milton Park, Abingdon, Oxon, OX14 4RN

PUBLISHER'S NOTE
The development, preparation, and publication of this work has been undertaken with great care. However, the Publisher, employees, editors, and agents of The Haworth Press are not responsible for any errors contained herein or for consequences that may ensue from use of materials or information contained in this work. The Haworth Press is committed to the dissemination of ideas and information according to the highest standards of intellectual freedom and the free exchange of ideas. Statements made and opinions expressed in this publication do not necessarily reflect the views of the Publisher, Directors, management, or staff of The Haworth Press, Inc., or an endorsement by them.

Front cover photograph of Dr. H. Anonymous (John E. Fryer, MD) by Kay Tobin Lahusen.

Library of Congress Cataloging-in-Publication Data

American psychiatry and homosexuality : an oral history / Jack Drescher, Joseph P. Merlino, editors
p. cm.
ISBN: 978-1-56023-738-9 (hard : alk. paper)
ISBN: 978-1-56023-739-6 (soft: alk. paper)
1. Homosexuality—Classification. 2. Homosexuality—United States—History. 3. Gay psychiatrists—United States—Interviews. 4. Diagnostic and statistical manual of mental disorders—History. 5. American Psychiatric Association—History. 6. Psychiatry—United States—History. I. Drescher, Jack, 1951- II. Merlino, Joseph P.
[DNLM: 1. American Psychiatric Association. 2. Psychiatry—United States—Interview. 3. Psychiatry—history—United States—Interview. 4. History, 20th Century—United States—Interview. 5. Homosexuality—United States—Interview. 6. Societies, Medical—United States—Interview. WM 11 AA1 A5125 2007]

RC558.A44 2007
616.89'008664—dc22

2007007020

Bertram Schaffner, MD, has played an immeasurable role in our personal and professional development. We dedicate this book to Bert, our friend, our mentor, and our family.

CONTENTS

SECTION II: THE EARLY FOUNDERS OF AGLP

SECTION III: GAY AND LESBIAN PSYCHIATRISTS OF NOTE

ABOUT THE EDITORS

Jack Drescher, MD, is a Fellow, Training and Supervising Analyst at the William Alanson White Institute and Adjunct Assistant Professor at New York University's Postdoctoral Program in Psychotherapy and Psychoanalysis. He is a Distinguished Fellow of the American Psychiatric Association and Past Chair (2000-2006) of its Committee on GLB Issues, as well as a Past President of APA's New York County District Branch. Dr. Drescher is the author of *Psychoanalytic Therapy and the Gay Man* (The Analytic Press) and editor of a score of books dealing with gender, sexuality, and public health. He is Editor-in-Chief of the *Journal of Gay and Lesbian Psychotherapy*™ (Haworth) and editor of the Bending Psychoanalysis Book Series (The Analytic Press). Dr. Drescher is in private practice in New York City.

Joseph P. Merlino, MD, MPA, is Director of Psychiatry at Queens Hospital Center in New York. He is Clinical Professor of Psychiatry at the Mt. Sinai School of Medicine and Adjunct Professor of Psychiatry and Behavioral Sciences at New York Medical College, where he is also a Training and Supervising Analyst. Dr. Merlino is a Distinguished Fellow of the American Psychiatric Association, a Fellow and Past President of the Academy of Psychoanalysis and Dynamic Psychiatry, and is an active member of the Group for the Advancement of Psychiatry and the American College of Psychiatrists. Dr. Merlino has written and lectured on the areas of applied psychoanalysis and health care ethics. He is in private practice in Manhattan.

American Psychiatry and Homosexuality: An Oral History

doi:10.1300/6049_a

Contributors

Kenn Ashley, MD, is Attending Psychiatrist, Beth Israel Medical Center, Department of Psychiatry, and Clinical Instructor, Department of Psychiatry, New York University School of Medicine, in New York City.

Mary E. Barber, MD, is Associate Medical Director at the Ulster County Mental Health Department in Kingston, New York, and President of the Association of Gay and Lesbian Psychiatrists.

Barbara Gittings was an early gay and lesbian rights activist, found of the New York City Chapter of the Daughters of Bilitis, and one of the individuals responsible for peruading the American Psychiatric Association to reconsider the diagnostic status of homosexuality in APA's *Diagnostic and Statistical Manual of Mental Disorders* (DSM). Her activities ultimately led to the 1973 APA decision to remove "homosexuality" from the DSM.

Richard O. Hire, MD, is Book Review Editor, *Journal of Gay & Lesbian Psychotherapy.* He is in private practice in New York City.

Joyce Hunter, DSW, is Co-Director of the Community Collaboration Core at the HIV Center for Clinical and Behavioral Studies, New York State Psychiatric Institute, in New York City.

Paul E. Lynch, MD, is Clinical Instructor in Psychiatry at Harvard University and the first openly gay candidate admitted to the Boston Psychoanalytic Institute. He is in private practice in Boston, Massachusetts.

Robert Mitchell, MD, is Assistant Clinical Professor of Psychiatry, New York University School of Medicine, and in private practice, in New York City.

American Psychiatry and Homosexuality: An Oral History

doi:10.1300/6049_b

Vernon A. Rosario, MD, PhD, is Child Psychiatry Fellow and Clinical Instructor at the UCLA Neuropsychiatric Institute in Los Angeles, California.

Albert J. Sbordone, MSW, PhD, is Clinical Adjunct, City University of New York, Doctoral Program in Clinical Psychology, and is in private practice in New York City.

David L. Scasta, MD, is Clinical Associate Professor of Psychiatry, Temple University Medical School, Philadelphia, Pennsylvania. He is in private practice in Forensics in Princeton, New Jersey.

Preface: Show-and-Tell

Barbara Gittings

When our American movement for full civil rights and equality for homosexuals got launched fifty-six years ago, we had a huge range of basic problems to tackle. We were denounced as immoral and sinful. We were punished as criminals and lawbreakers. We were labeled "sick" and needing a "cure." We were mostly invisible as gay, which made it hard for gay men and lesbians to develop good social lives and to create a movement to battle injustice and prejudice.

It's difficult to explain to anyone who didn't live through that time how much homosexuality was under the thumb of psychiatry. The sickness label was an albatross around the neck of our early gay rights groups—it infected all our work on other issues. Anything we said on our behalf could be dismissed as "That's just your sickness talking." The sickness label was used to justify discrimination, especially in employment, and especially by our own government.

Some brutal methods for curing us in vogue at one time included incarceration in mental hospitals, lobotomies, and aversion therapy. The latter is where they show you pictures of the "wrong" kind of sexual partner and give you an electric shock, and then show you pictures of a person you *should* like and play nice music to persuade you to change your choice of sexual partner.

There were of course other efforts at curing homosexuality that were less physically brutal, including psychotherapy, but they all thrived on the notion that homosexuality was bad for the individual

---

This chapter was delivered upon Barbara Gittings' accepting the American Psychiatric Association's first John E. Fryer, MD Award. The award is for a public figure who has made significant contributions to LGBT mental health and was given on October 7, 2006, in New York City at APA's 58th Institute on Psychiatric Services.

American Psychiatry and Homosexuality: An Oral History

doi:10.1300/6049_c

and for society and should be fixed. You can see more on this in a documentary video called *One Nation Under God.* Though the film is mainly about the faith ministries that try to convert gays to heterosexuality, it's chock full of anecdotes on psychiatric cures and footage of psychiatrists expounding on how sick homosexuals are.

You all know about one book that especially popularized the sickness view. *Homosexuality: A Psychoanalytic Study,* published in 1962, claimed to be a scientific study comparing a group of gay men in psychoanalysis with a group of heterosexual men also in analysis.[1] The authors, including Dr. Irving Bieber, pumped in at the beginning their belief that homosexuality was psychopathological, and they worked their meager statistics up and down and sideways, and lo! At the end they plucked out those beliefs as scientific conclusions.

What a shameful work. More shameful is that it was uncritically accepted at the time. I'm not aware of a single review or comment in the contemporary psychiatric literature that pointed out that the Bieber authors failed to follow science. This bothered me. I talked to a psychologist, Dr. Fritz Fluckiger. He wrote a detailed critique of the Bieber study called "Research Through a Glass, Darkly." It was published in 1966 in *The Ladder,* the magazine of the national lesbian organization the Daughters of Bilitis, which I was editing at the time. Unfortunately Dr. Fluckiger wasn't an MD analyst and his review wasn't published in a professional journal.

But reaction was building to the sickness label's bad effect on gay individuals' self-image and on our movement's fight for equality. One of the psychoanalysts who participated in the Bieber study gave a public lecture in December 1964 plainly titled "Homosexuality: A Disease." Four gay protesters showed up; they demanded and got ten minutes of rebuttal time for their spokesman.

Another key event was the antisickness statement adopted in 1965 by the Mattachine Society of Washington, DC, and many other gay organizations. Eventually gay groups were demanding official reconsideration of homosexuality as sickness. A petition to the American Psychiatric Association (APA) appeared in a lesbian newspaper in 1971. We were also taking a proactive stand, saying, "We Are the Experts on Homosexuality."

Changes in thinking were brewing among psychiatrists, spurred in part by the pioneer work in the 1950s of psychologist Dr. Evelyn Hooker, which challenged traditional views about homosexuality.[2]

Psychiatrist Dr. Judd Marmor was especially influential because of his own evolution away from the old orthodoxy.[3] A good account of the developing shift is in Ronald Bayer's book *Homosexuality and American Psychiatry: The Politics of Diagnosis,* published in 1981.[4]

Things came to a head in 1970 when gays invaded several psychiatric meetings, targeting in particular sessions on aversion therapy. Protesters seized microphones and denounced psychiatry for hurting instead of helping us. The angry disrupters said, "Stop talking about us and start talking with us."

Wisely, the APA met this demand. At its 1971 meeting in Washington, DC, there was a panel of gay people including Frank Kameny titled "Lifestyles of Non-Patient Homosexuals." We jokingly called it "Lifestyles of Impatient Homosexuals." But it was the first time the APA acknowledged that there are homosexuals who aren't in therapy and have no need for it.

Also Frank and I disrupted a lecture on aversion therapy and forced an exhibitor of aversion therapy materials to remove the slides he was selling for use on homosexuals.

The next year, 1972, Frank and I were invited to be on a panel in Dallas called "Psychiatry: Friend or Foe to Homosexuals—A Dialogue." My partner Kay said, "This isn't right. Here you have two psychiatrists pitted against two gays, and what you really need is someone who is both." The panel moderator, Dr. Kent Robinson, agreed to add a gay psychiatrist if we could find one. In 1972, who would come forward? Oh, how we searched! Kay and I wrote letters and made phone calls around the country. (Remember, no e-mail in those days.)

At last, John Fryer said yes, provided he could wear a wig and mask and use a voice-distorting microphone. Dr. H. Anonymous was born.[5]

We smuggled him in his disguise through back corridors into the packed lecture hall. He really rocked the audience, speaking as a closeted gay person to his own colleagues, telling why he couldn't be open in his own profession. To back up John Fryer, I read excerpts from letters I'd solicited from the other gay psychiatrists who felt they had to decline to be on the panel.

Also at the 1972 APA meeting, Frank and I were given a booth in the exhibit hall. With much help from friends, I set up an eye-grabbing display, "Gay, Proud, and Healthy: The Homosexual Community Speaks." Frank wrote the flyer. This exhibit featured the word LOVE in big letters. I think it was the *only* place in the whole convention where that word LOVE appeared.

There were more eye-openers for the psychiatrists. At APA's dinner-dance, at the conclusion of the conference, Frank took as his date Philip Johnson, a gay activist from Dallas. And when the band struck up a waltz, Frank and Phil sailed out onto the dance floor. The other heterosexual dance couples all pretended they didn't see what they saw!

Meanwhile, behind the scenes in APA, the wheels were already moving to consider taking homosexuality off the list of mental disorders as part of a general revision of the *Diagnostic and Statistical Manual*.[6] This long and difficult debate is well recounted in Bayer's book. When the Board of Trustees endorsed the recommendation to delist homosexuality in December 1973, a major Philadelphia newspaper headlined its story "Homosexuals Gain 'Instant Cure.'" The trustees also passed a civil rights resolution opposing laws and official discrimination against gay people.[7]

Of course a stroke of the pen doesn't change attitudes. Objections to the "official cure" were contested by psychiatrists who petitioned for a referendum of APA membership that took place in 1974. This political battle is told in detail in Bayer's book *Homosexuality and American Psychiatry.*

Mindful of the need for continuing education, APA gave the National Gay and Lesbian Task Force exhibit space at several later conventions. In 1976, in Miami, we did "Homophobia: Time for Cure," with displays of materials illustrating anti-gay attitudes and policies and practices. Part of our prescription to cure homophobia included photos of gay couples. Surprisingly, they drew strong reaction. One dubious doctor asked, "Do these relationships really work?" Many psychiatrists were used to thinking of us as miserable patients with troubled lives, and they needed to see some reality.

At this time, 1976, gay psychiatrists were coming out of the closet and had launched a GLB Caucus, whose newsletter was on hand. Its members helped staff the booth to talk to colleagues.

My last APA exhibit, "Gay Love: Good Medicine," was in Atlanta in 1978. Again we featured gays not as patients but living happy and healthy. And this time I was able to get five gay psychiatrists willing to be in the exhibit with their photos and credentials—quite a breakthrough! The GLB Caucus in APA was now taking steps to become an official subgroup of APA.[8]

Still the closet was emptying slowly. One psychiatrist wrote the piece "The Invisible Gay Psychiatrist" for distribution at that 1978 conference; he urged those who couldn't come out to take other specific steps to push things along.

By 1979, the GLB Caucus went fully public by taking part in the gay community's first National March on Washington. You know well the rest of your history.

I am thankful to the American Psychiatric Association and to the Association of Gay and Lesbian Psychiatrists for recognizing my and Frank Kameny's work toward healing the wounds of prejudice and discrimination. I'm sure John Fryer would be thrilled and deeply gratified, as I am, for having an APA award presented in his name and for the first one going to Frank and myself. By drawing attention to the mask and the damage it does, Dr. H. Anonymous helped tear away disguise and secrecy. He gave courage to his fellow gay and lesbian psychiatrists to be fully themselves and to affirm, in Frank's great motto, that Gay Is Good.

The gay community's mental health improved dramatically when we spoke up for ourselves and took charge of our own destiny. I'm so glad I was a player in this part of gay history and that I got to know the incomparable John Fryer.

NOTES

1. Bieber, I., Dain, H.J., Dince, P.R., Drellich, M.G., Grand, H.G., Gundlach, R.H., Kremer, M.W., Rifkin, A.H., Wilbur, C.B. & Bieber T.B. (1962), *Homosexuality: A Psychoanalytic Study.* New York: Basic Books.

2. Hooker, E.A. (1957), The adjustment of the male overt homosexual. *J. Projective Techniques,* 21:18-31.

3. Marmor, J., ed. (1965), *Sexual Inversion: The Multiple Roots of Homosexuality.* New York: Basic Books. Also see Veron Rosario's interview with Judd Marmor, MD, Chapter 5 in this book.

4. Bayer, R. (1981), *Homosexuality and American Psychiatry: The Politics of Diagnosis.* New York: Basic Books.

5. See David Scasta's article on John E. Fryer, MD, and the Dr. H. Anonymous episode, Chapter 1 in this book.

6. See Jack Drescher's interview with Robert L. Spitzer, MD, Chapter 6 in this book; Albert Sbordone's interview with Charles Silverstein, PhD, Chapter 2 in this

book; and Richard Hire's interview with Robert Jean Campbell III, MD, Chapter 4 in this book.

7. "Whereas homosexuality in and of itself implies no impairment in judgment, stability, reliability, or vocational capabilities, therefore, be it resolved that the American Psychiatric Association deplores all public and private discrimination against homosexuals in such areas as employment, housing, public accommodations, and licensing, and declares that no burden of proof of such judgment, capacity, or reliability shall be placed on homosexuals greater than that imposed on any other persons. Further, the APA supports and urges the enactment of civil rights legislation at local, state, and federal levels that would insure homosexual citizens the same protections now guaranteed to others. Further, the APA supports and urges the repeal of all legislation making criminal offenses of sexual acts performed by consenting adults in private." Retrieved from http://www.psych.org/edu/other_res/lib_archives/archives/197310.pdf#search=%22homosexuality%22.

8. See Richard Hire's interview with Frank Rundle, MD, Chapter 7 in this book; Kenn Ashley's interview with Stuart E. Nichols, MD, Chapter 10 in this book; and Mary Barber's interviews with Nanette Gartrell, MD, and David E. Kessler, MD, Chapters 9 and 8, respectively, in this book.

Introduction

Jack Drescher
Joseph P. Merlino

As years go, 1973 was one for the history books. The World Trade Center officially opened. The U.S. Supreme Court decided *Roe v. Wade* and overturned state bans on abortions. The United States began ending its involvement in the Vietnam War. The cold war was in full chill, and to maintain the balance of power, Communist East Germany and democratic West Germany were simultaneously admitted to the United Nations. The democratically elected, leftist government of Salvador Allende was violently overthrown, with U.S. backing, in a military coup. Israel fought Egypt and Syria in the Yom Kippur War, leading to an Arab oil embargo and a global energy crisis. The Watergate scandal led to calls for President Richard Nixon's impeachment and Vice President Spiro Agnew resigned his office following charges of tax evasion.

Then, if all that was not enough, on December 15, 1973, the Board of Trustees of the American Psychiatric Association (APA) voted to remove homosexuality from their *Diagnostic and Statistical Manual of Mental Disorders* (DSM).

What led the APA to stop the psychiatric pathologizing of homosexuality that had begun with nineteenth-century degeneracy theory (Krafft-Ebing, 1886) and was later taken up by twentieth-century ego psychology is explored in this volume through the personal back stories of many of the individuals involved.

Before 1973, homosexuality per se was classified as an "antisocial" disorder in APA's first edition of the *Diagnostic and Statistical Manual* (DSM-I) (APA, 1952) and as a "perversion" in DSM-II (APA, 1968). Although some psychiatrists of that time—including the late Judd Marmor (profiled in this volume)—did not believe homosexuality to be pathological, this was a minority viewpoint. Amer-

American Psychiatry and Homosexuality: An Oral History

doi:10.1300/6049_01

ican psychiatry, influenced at the time by psychoanalytic "ego psychology," mostly ignored a growing body of sexology research and its normalizing conclusions about homosexuality. Significant studies included the 1948 and 1953 Kinsey reports and Evelyn Hooker's 1957 study, which showed that nonpathological expressions of homosexuality were common. However, as a conservative, medical organization, APA was not initially receptive to studying the validity of scientific research done in other fields, particularly since those nonpsychiatric studies were critical of the psychiatric theory and practice of the time. However, in 1970 this research was brought forcefully to the attention of the APA.

In the wake of 1969's Stonewall riots in New York City's Greenwich Village, a modern gay and lesbian civil rights movement emerged (Duberman, 1994). Organized gay activists, convinced that psychiatry's pathologizing attitudes about homosexuality were a major contributor to social stigma, disrupted first the 1970 and then again the 1971 annual APA meetings. In response to these protests, the APA permitted two educational panels at the 1971 and 1972 meetings. The 1971 panel, titled "Lifestyles of Non-Patient Homosexuals," featured non-patient gay activists explaining to their psychiatric audience the stigma caused by the "homosexuality" diagnosis (see Barbara Gittings' preface, in this volume).

At the 1972 meeting, the activists returned for another panel, "Psychiatry: Friend or Foe to Homosexuals—A Dialogue." However, this time they were joined by a psychiatrist, John Fryer, MD (also profiled in this volume), who appeared as "Dr. H. Anonymous." Fryer disguised his true identity from the audience and spoke of the discrimination gay psychiatrists faced in their own profession. As an openly gay physician could lose his medical license at that time, Fryer wore a rubber mask, a fright wig, and an oversized tuxedo. He told his audience in a disguised voice:

> As psychiatrists who are homosexual, we must know our place and what we must do to be successful. If our goal is academic appointment, a level of earning capacity equal to our fellows, or admission to a psychoanalytic institute, we must make certain that no one in a position of power is aware of our sexual orientation or gender identity. Much like the black man with the light skin who chooses to live as a white man, we cannot be seen with our real friends—our real homosexual family—lest our secret

be known and our dooms sealed. (see Chapter 1 in this book, p. 23)

During the time these public panels were going on, the APA had also embarked upon an internal process of studying the scientific question of whether homosexuality should be considered a psychiatric disorder. APA's Nomenclature Committee was the scientific body charged with addressing this issue. Under the leadership of Robert Spitzer, MD (also profiled in this volume), the committee reviewed the psychiatric and psychoanalytic literature on the subject as well as the sexology literature. The latter, a subject not usually taught in psychiatric training programs at that time, was unfamiliar to most practicing psychiatrists.

Following their study of the issue, the APA Nomenclature Committee recommended removing homosexuality per se from the diagnostic manual. After review and approval by other APA committees and deliberative bodies, in December 1973, APA's Board of Trustees voted to remove homosexuality from the DSM. This marked the end of the classification of homosexuality per se as an illness. Within two

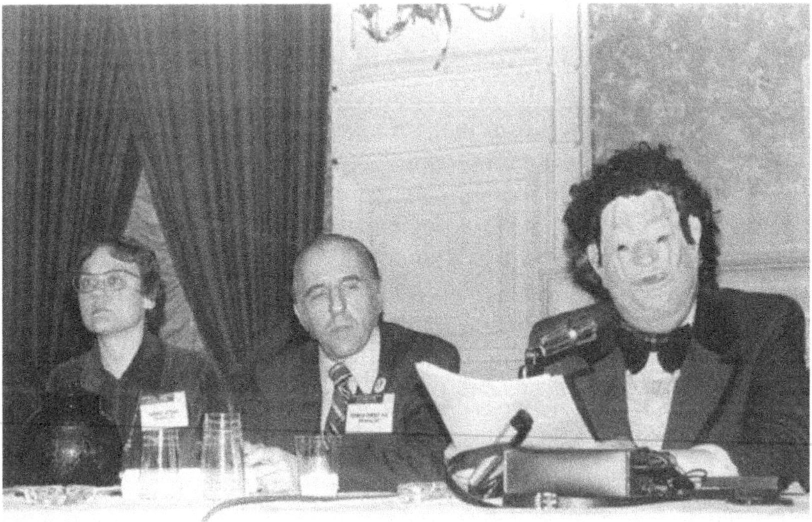

Barbara Gittings, Frank Kameny, and Dr. H. Anonymous (John Fryer, MD). Photograph by Kay Tobin Lahusen.

years, other major mental health professional organizations, including the American Psychological Association, the National Association of Social Workers, and the Association for Advancement of Behavior Therapy, endorsed the APA decision.

However, psychiatrists who objected to the removal, mostly among the psychoanalytic community, petitioned to have a referendum in which the entire APA membership could vote on the issue (Bayer, 1981). In 1974, the decision to remove was upheld by a 58 percent majority of voting members. The APA also issued a groundbreaking position statement supporting civil rights protection for gay people:

> Whereas homosexuality in and of itself implies no impairment in judgment, stability, reliability, or vocational capabilities, therefore, be it resolved that the American Psychiatric Association deplores all public and private discrimination against homosexuals in such areas as employment, housing, public accommodations, and licensing, and declares that no burden of proof of such judgment, capacity, or reliability shall be placed on homosexuals greater than that imposed on any other persons. Further, the APA supports and urges the enactment of civil rights legislation at local, state, and federal levels that would insure homosexual citizens the same protections now guaranteed to others. Further, the APA supports and urges the repeal of all legislation making criminal offenses of sexual acts performed by consenting adults in private.[1]

The APA nosology, with a focus on evidence-based medicine, would eventually create a new standard for diagnosis in the international psychiatric community. Consequently, in 1992, the World Health Organization (WHO) accepted APA's view and removed the diagnosis of homosexuality per se from the tenth edition of the *International Classification of Diseases* (ICD-10) (WHO, 1992a,b; also see Nakajima, 2003).

Many consider Ronald Bayer's (1981) *Homosexuality and American Psychiatry: The Politics of Diagnosis* to be one of the most important chronicles of the history just outlined. However, Bayer, in his analysis of the 1973 APA decision, concluded it was unlikely that psychiatry had the power to take the lead in changing society's attitudes toward homosexuality. He maintained that

> the psychiatric mainstream must ultimately affirm the standards of health and disease of the society within which it works. It cannot hold to discordant views regarding the normal and abnormal, the desirable and undesirable, and continue to perform its socially sanctioned function. (p. 194)

However, Bayer's conclusions, published only eight years after the APA decision, have not been borne out. Since the APA decision, and particularly in the last decade, there has been an unprecedented social acceptance of gay men and women in both public and private arenas that was unimaginable during the era when homosexuality was considered a psychiatric illness. In fact, as in the biblical story of the ancient Hebrews who fled from Egypt and who were forced to wander in the desert, it appears that an entire generation had to die out before the next one could enter the Promised Land.[2]

This brings us to this *Oral History,* which began as a series of profiles that were published individually in the *Journal of Gay & Lesbian Psychotherapy* between 2001 and 2006. Seventeen profiles are gathered here together to supplement existing scholarship of the events surrounding the 1973 decision and to illustrate some of the consequences that changes in psychiatric nosology have had, both in American psychiatry and in the culture at large.

We wish to note with great sadness that three of the individuals interviewed since we began this profiles project have passed on: Stu Nichols, Frank Rundle, and Judd Marmor. We also mourn the loss of our friend and collaborator, Richard Hire, who died in 2005.

We have organized the profiles into three sections. The first includes interviews of individuals (not all of whom were psychiatrists and not all of whom were gay) who had some role to play in the APA decision to remove homosexuality from DSM-II. The second section features psychiatrists who, following the events of 1973, played an important role in organizing gay, lesbian, and bisexual (GLB) psychiatrists within the APA and later in the founding of the Association of Gay and Lesbian Psychiatrists (AGLP). The third section profiles some of the psychiatrists who have made important contributions, not only to the GLB psychiatric community, but to the psychiatric and mental health mainstream as well. There are many other GLBT psychiatrists who are worthy of being similarly profiled and we hope that the *JGLP* will do so in the future.

Section I begins with David Scasta's profile of John Fryer, MD. Dr. Fryer, who died in 2003, was a child prodigy whose iconoclasm came early and easily; his willingness to test boundaries was both his genius and frequently his undoing. Yet, as mentioned earlier, this colorful and perpetually controversial man had the right talent at the right time to become a pivotal figure in the historical battle for gay liberation. In this profile he details his participation at the May 1972 APA annual meeting where he appeared before the world as Dr. H. Anonymous.

Charles Silverstein, PhD, saw the diagnosis of homosexuality as a means of social control that kept gay people feeling ashamed, in a state of low self-esteem, and often depressed. In this state, he argued, many gay people sought the help of therapists, to try to become heterosexual. Silverstein, profiled by Albert Sbordone, spoke from personal experience; years before the 1973 decision, when consulting with his first psychoanalyst, he wanted to change into a heterosexual; and if the analyst would not help him do so, Silverstein would not see him. When the APA's Nomenclature Committee convened to consider the issue of homosexuality's diagnostic status on February 8, 1973, Silverstein, who was still working on his doctoral dissertation in psychology at the time, presented what turned out to be compelling arguments in favor of removal.

Lawrence Hartmann, MD's parents were both psychiatrists. His father, Heinz Hartmann, along with Anna Freud, is considered one of the major theorists of psychoanalytic ego psychology. For a variety of reasons, including the fact that he was gay, Hartmann chose not to seek formal psychoanalytic training for himself. His interests in dynamic and social psychiatry, in biopsychosocial integration, in the plight of women, children, and minorities, in homosexuality and in human rights issues have led him to much activity and several leadership positions in both child and adult psychiatric organizations. In this profile by Jack Drescher, he recounts his early efforts to help reform the American Psychiatric Association, and his role in removing homosexuality from the DSM. Hartmann would go on to become President of the American Psychiatric Association from 1991-1992.

Robert J. Campbell, MD, was a member of the APA Nomenclature Committee during the period prior to the 1973 decision. In this profile by the late Richard Hire, he tells of his role in persuading that committee to allow a presentation of scientific data by the gay activists.

He also suggested that the committee create a task force, which would be chaired by Robert Spitzer, to research the matter further. Campbell went on to a remarkable career in the American Psychiatric Association, was Vice President of APA, and was nominated twice for APA President.

Judd Marmor, MD, is profiled by Vernon Rosario. Marmor, who died in 2004, was an early psychoanalytic critic of theories that pathologized homosexuality (Marmor, 1965). A heterosexual ally of GLB psychiatrists, he was tireless in his support of fairness and equality. He participated in the panel with Dr. H. Anonymous. Marmor played an important leadership role in American psychiatry, not only during the 1973 decision, but also serving as President of the American Psychiatric Association, the American Academy of Psychoanalysis, and the Group for the Advancement of Psychiatry.

Robert Spitzer, MD, chaired the subcommittee of the Nomenclature Committee that recommended the removal of homosexuality from the DSM to the APA Board of Trustees. Spitzer is also considered the "father" of modern psychiatric nosology thanks to his efforts in shaping the DSM-III. In his profile by Jack Drescher, Spitzer recounts his role in the 1973 decision as well as some commentary on his 2003 study of ex-gays and its impact on the culture wars (also see Drescher and Zucker, 2006).

Section II focuses on psychiatrists who, following the removal of homosexuality from the DSM, began the process of creating a normalizing presence of GLB psychiatrists within the APA and who went on to organize the Association of Gay and Lesbian Psychiatrists (AGLP). Frank Rundle, MD, like many gay men of his time, got married and had children before he eventually came out as a gay man. In 1978, at the APA meeting in Atlanta, he helped organize the first gathering of what would later become the APA Caucus of Gay, Lesbian, and Bisexual Psychiatrists. In this profile by Richard Hire, he tells of the continuing opposition within APA, six years after the 1973 decision, to greater inclusiveness. Rundle, who died in 2004, was the first President of the APA's GLB Caucus (which would later grow into AGLP) from 1977-1980.

David Kessler, MD, is profiled by Mary Barber. Kessler was AGLP President from 1980-1982. He has endowed the David R. Kessler lectures in Lesbian and Gay Studies at the Center for Lesbian and Gay Studies (CLAGS) of the City University of New York. This series, the first of its kind at an academic institution, has honored prominent figures in the lesbian and gay community with an annual lecture since its inception in 1992. Past honorees have included Edmund White, Judith Butler, Samuel Delany, Eve Kosofsky Sedgwick, and John D'Emilio. The first ten Kessler lectures have been published as a book (CLAGS, 2003).

Nanette Gartrell, MD, also profiled by Mary Barber, was both an early woman member of AGLP and a pioneer for feminist issues within the American Psychiatric Association. Her National Longitudinal Lesbian Family Study has been in progress since 1986, in an effort to shed light on the lives of lesbian mothers and their children. Gartrell was the first "out" lesbian on the Harvard Medical School faculty.

Stuart Nichols, MD, died in 2002. In addition to being President of AGLP from 1983-1984, in 1978 Nichols was a founding member of Gay and Lesbian Psychiatrists of New York (GLPNY) and its first President from 1978-1980. Nichols was also a founding member of both the American Association of Physicians for Human Rights—now known as the Gay and Lesbian Medical Association (GLMA)—and the New York Physicians for Human Rights, now known as New York Gay and Lesbian Physicians (NYGLP). His profile is by Kenn Ashley.

Emery Hetrick, MD, died in 1986, more than a decade before we began the *JGLP* profile series. However, Emery's contributions to the GLB community were of such a magnitude, we invited his good friend Joyce Hunter to write a tribute to him. At the 1978 annual meeting of the APA, a photo of Emery as an openly gay psychiatrist, with his partner, Damien Martin, PhD, was displayed at a booth in the exhibition hall that featured the theme "Gay Love: Good Medicine." Emery was an energetic founding member of both AGLP and GLPNY. Emery was also a cofounder and supporter of Senior Action in a Gay Environment (SAGE), a group providing social support and social services in New York. In 1979, Emery and Damien formed an education and advocacy group, the Institute for the Protection of Lesbian and Gay Youth, which would eventually house the internationally famous Harvey Milk School. After their deaths in the 1980s, the institute was named after its founders as the Hetrick-Martin Institute.

Section III, the final section of interviews, focuses on gay and lesbian psychiatrists making contributions to the mental health fields.

Bertram Schaffner, MD, was our first choice to initiate the profile series project in the *JGLP,* and it is to Dr. Schaffner that this book is dedicated. At the end of World War II, at the suggestion of Margaret Mead, he worked on the denazification process in occupied Germany and wrote the book *Fatherland: A Study of Authoritarianism in the German Family,* published in 1948 with a preface by Margaret Mead. From 1948 to 1962, he brought together various groups from West Indian islands, to form the U.S. Caribbean Aid to Mental Health, of which he was Executive Director and fund-raiser for many years. From the onset of the AIDS epidemic, Dr. Schaffner has been on the front lines caring for patients and caregivers. He was instrumental in providing group psychotherapy for physicians with AIDS (along with Stu Nichols until his death) from 1985 until the present time. The profile is by Joseph P. Merlino.

Martha Kirkpatrick, MD, has been a longtime leader in psychiatry and psychoanalysis, both as a woman and an "out" lesbian. As a dedicated, challenging, and much sought-after supervisor, Kirkpatrick has mentored numerous psychoanalysts and psychiatrists in Los Angeles. She has particularly been a mentor to a long line of gay psychiatry residents, including her interviewer, Vernon Rosario. She has published extensively on the psychodynamics of female sexuality, psychotherapy with lesbians, and lesbian parenting.

Richard Isay, MD, is interviewed by Robert Mitchell. Isay is known to many as the first openly gay psychoanalyst in the American Psychoanalytic Association (APsaA). Among his many important clinical contributions to psychiatry and psychoanalysis is his developmental theory for male homosexuality, a major revision of the classical psychoanalytic theory. He also played a decisive role in making it possible for openly gay men and women to be accepted for analytic training in the institutes of the APsaA.

Richard Pillard, MD, is best known for studying the incidence of homosexuality in families and twins, and reporting the evidence for genetic heritability. Pillard, who is profiled by Paul Lynch, has authored about 100 book chapters, articles, reviews, posters, and editorials on psychopharmacology, sexual orientation, and the genetics of deafness. He was also the founder of one of the first gay-oriented health services in the United States: The Homophile Community Health Service in Boston, Massachusetts.

Edward Hanin, MD, has had an outstanding and distinguished career in American psychiatry, and particularly within the APA, where he has served in many important positions, most notably as Speaker of the APA Assembly from 1990-1991. Hanin, interviewed by Jack Drescher, has been the recipient of numerous professional awards, including the New York State Psychiatric Association's George L. Ginsberg, MD Award, the APA Assembly's Award for Meritorious Service, and the APA's Warren Williams, MD Award.

We conclude with Paul Lynch's profile of Ralph Roughton, MD, a Training and Supervising Psychoanalyst at the Emory University Psychoanalytic Institute. In 1991, Roughton was appointed the first Chair of the APsaA's Committee on Gay, Lesbian, and Bisexual Issues. In this role, he spoke at psychoanalytic institutes across the United States, acted as a consultant to the institutes, and spoke frequently and frankly at the meetings of the APsaA. In doing so, Roughton helped broaden and personalize discussions of homosexuality among American psychoanalysts. When he came out of the closet in 1996, Roughton became the first openly gay Training and Supervising Psychoanalyst to be recognized within the American and International Psychoanalytic Associations. To acknowledge his achievements, the APsaA now offers an annual "Ralph Roughton Award for Outstanding Contributions to the Literature on Homosexuality" in his honor.

NOTES

1. http://www.psych.org/edu/other_res/lib_archives/archives/197310.pdf#search=%22homosexuality%22.
2. See Numbers XIV.

REFERENCES

American Psychiatric Association (1952), *Diagnostic and Statistical Manual of Mental Disorders.* Washington, DC: American Psychiatric Association.

American Psychiatric Association (1968), *Diagnostic and Statistical Manual of Mental Disorders,* Second Edition. Washington, DC: American Psychiatric Press.

American Psychiatric Association (1980), *Diagnostic and Statistical Manual of Mental Disorders,* Third Edition. Washington, DC: American Psychiatric Press.

Bayer, R. (1981), *Homosexuality and American Psychiatry: The Politics of Diagnosis.* New York: Basic Books.

CLAGS (2003), *Queer Ideas: The David R. Kessler Lectures in Lesbian and Gay Studies.* New York: Feminist Press.

Drescher, J. & Zucker, K.J., eds. (2006), *Ex-Gay Research: Analyzing the Spitzer Study and Its Relation to Science, Religion, Politics, and Culture.* Binghamton, NY: The Haworth Press.

Duberman, M. (1994), *Stonewall.* New York: Plume.

Hooker, E.A. (1957), The adjustment of the male overt homosexual. *J. Projective Techniques,* 21:18-31.

Kinsey, A.C., Pomeroy, W.B. & Martin C.E. (1948), *Sexual Behavior in the Human Male.* Philadelphia, PA: W.B. Saunders.

Kinsey, A., Pomeroy, W., Martin, C. & Gebhard, P. (1953), *Sexual Behavior in the Human Female.* Philadelphia, PA: W.B. Saunders.

Krafft-Ebing, R. (1886), *Psychopathia Sexualis,* trans. H. Wedeck. New York: Putnam, 1965.

Marmor, J., ed. (1965), *Sexual Inversion: The Multiple Roots of Homosexuality.* New York: Basic Books.

Nakajima, G.A. (2003), The emergence of an international lesbian, gay, and bisexual psychiatric movement. *J. Gay & Lesbian Psychotherapy,* 7(1/2):165-188. Reprinted in: *The Mental Health Professions and Homosexuality: International Perspectives,* ed. V. Lingiardi & J. Drescher. Binghamton, NY: The Haworth Press, 2003, pp. 165-188.

Schaffner, B. (1948), *Fatherland: A Study of Authoritarianism in the German Family.* New York: Columbia University Press.

World Health Organization (1992a), *The ICD-10 Classification of Mental and Behavioural Disorders: Clinical Descriptions and Diagnostic Guidelines.* Geneva, Switzerland: World Health Organization.

World Health Organization (1992b), *International Statistical Classification of Diseases and Health Related Problems,* Tenth Revision (ICD-10) (Vol. 1). Geneva, Switzerland: World Health Organization.

SECTION I:
THE 1973 APA DECISION

Chapter 1

John E. Fryer, MD, and the Dr. H. Anonymous Episode

David L. Scasta

Prologue

Nothing about John Fryer is subtle: a large man, six feet four inches tall with a weight that hovers around the 300 mark; with bulldog jowls and an impish smile that seems to suggest that he has just heard a most titillating secret about you; a man who can be witty and charming or petulant and biting; a man with a quick, intuitive sense of what others are feeling and, at other times, self-absorbed and entitled; a man as comfortable behind the ranks of the organ as he is as an orator about those matters for which he has passion; a man as much maligned for his display of sexual orientation as he is praised for his multiple talents; a man who stands a little too close and still harbors the wounds of disdain from those who never accepted him as he is and push him away. John was a child prodigy–an ingénue–whose iconoclasm came early and easily; whose willingness to test boundaries was both his genius and frequently his undoing. Yet, this colorful and perpetually controversial man had the right talent at the right time to become a pivotal figure in the battle for gay liberation. For years he has been known only as Dr. H. Anonymous. This is his story. The *Journal of Gay & Lesbian Psychotherapy* is pleased to provide him a place to tell it.

This chapter appeared originally under the same title in *Journal of Gay & Lesbian Psychotherapy* 6(4):73-84.

American Psychiatry and Homosexuality: An Oral History
Published by The Haworth Press, Inc., 2007.
doi:10.1300/6049_02

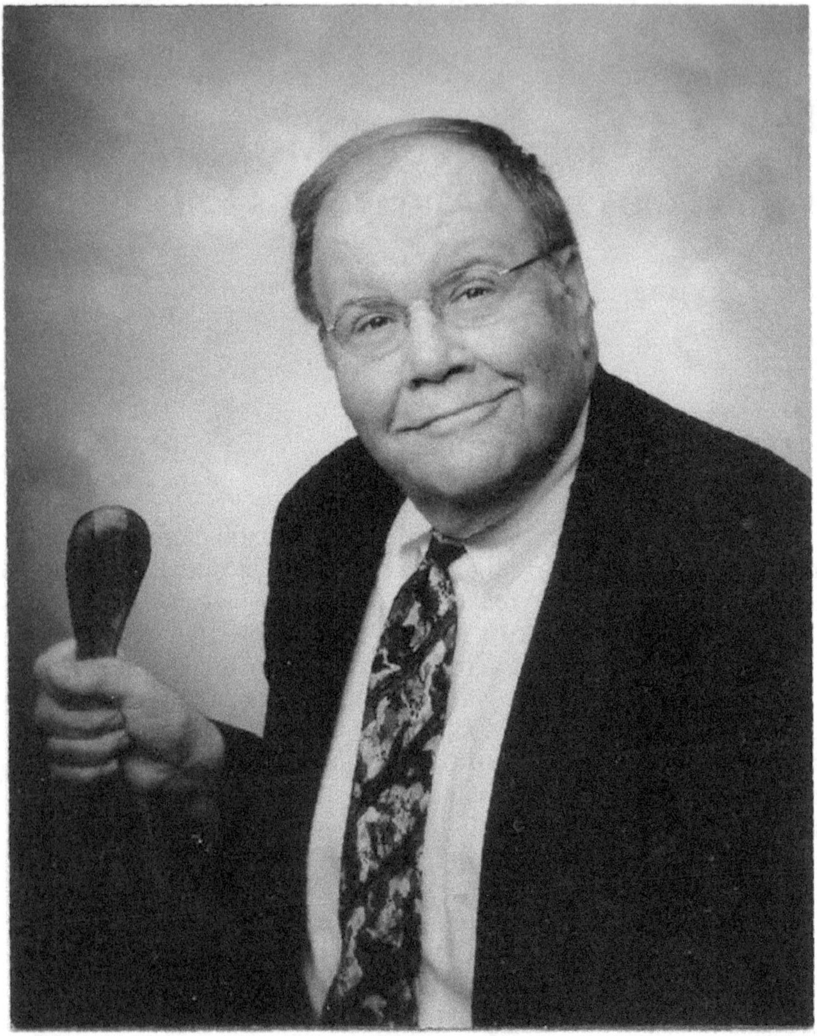

I entered second grade at age five, finished high school around age fifteen, went to Transylvania University in Kentucky, and by age nineteen was a first-year medical student at Vanderbilt University. I was fourteen when I did the "deed." It was on the way to band rehearsal. He was a sixteen-year-old jock who had a car and I rode with him to pick up some drums for the rehearsal. While we waited in the car for the drums to become available, he started feeling me up and asked me if I wanted "to do something." The drums interrupted the seduction until after band rehearsal when he made a point to insist that he would be taking me home. Instead, we went to the back of the local grade school, where we "did it." After that we continued to have sex. We had a lot of sex over the next several years. I still stay in touch with him. He went on to marry—several times.

I have always been drawn to a lot of people. There is this thing in the gay world where gays are encouraged to become like straight people—that is, marry and then play around on the edge of that marriage. In fact, my experience with the gay psychiatrists was that on the one hand they looked at me as kind of not normal because I wasn't bonded with one individual. On the other hand, what I found was that, whenever I brought one of my boyfriends to their meetings, he was hit on four or five times before we left by people who were ostensibly coupled. I didn't want to keep that kind of mythology alive by trying to live the heterosexual model. I am a very intense person and difficult to live with and I just didn't feel like I needed somebody all the time. Consequently, there has been this whole procession of people, many of whom I have been open and sexual with for twenty-five years. There is tremendous loyalty between them and me. I go and see them and they come and see me two and three times a year. To a large degree, that arrangement is just an extension of the way I was in college and medical school in that I had a lot of friends—a lot of people with whom I was sexual—and never really thought that I needed to "come out" because I always knew that I was gay and most of my close friends knew that I was gay. For many years, I was oblivious to that whole issue of coming out and was absorbed by frequent sexual rendezvous. But I get ahead of myself. It wasn't until my psychiatry residency that things changed.

I was very close to one medical student when I was in medical school—we had a lot of rotations together. During one of those rotations at the VA Hospital, our relationship became increasingly intense and began to have romantic overtones. He asked if he could come back to my room with me, to which I agreed. He then kissed me and said, "I know you want more, but I can't give it to you." It became clear to me that people saw me as gay. I didn't stand up and say I was gay. People just seemed to know it.

I did my first year of residency at Ohio State as a medicine intern. At that time, I did not come out to any of my superiors nor any of my colleagues. I then went to the Menninger Foundation in Topeka, Kansas, to begin my psychiatry residency while keeping my sexuality private. But when I went out to the gay bars in Topeka, I was always in danger of running into someone I knew. There were only 100,000 people in Topeka at that time and two-thirds of those were connected with the Menninger Foundation—either as a patient or an administrator or an employee. So I could be certain that if I did go to one of the gay bars in Topeka, I would run into somebody from the Menninger Foundation—and I did. As a result, I started going to Kansas City, Missouri, making a mad dash at eighty miles an hour, some sixty or seventy miles away. I think that that was the only highway in the country that at that time had an eighty-mile-per-hour speed limit.

There was a lot of homophobia at Menninger, making it very clear that coming out was not something that I could do. It was a situation in which I needed to be open as a psychiatrist-in-training but could not be because I did not trust people. Halfway through my first year, my supervisor noticed that I was very depressed and told me that, as a resident, the residency would pay for three free hours of psychoanalysis. He sent me to Dorothea Dana, an analyst. I felt that in that setting and in that place I could be honest with her, although I was apprehensive because everyone was in analysis. People who were my supervisors had been in analysis for eighteen to twenty years, and there were many people whom I knew at Topeka who had died still undergoing analysis. And that wasn't what I wanted. I was totally honest with her and I told her of my reservations. She replied in her German accent, "There is only one solution. Did you ever think of leaving Topeka?" That question was like a godsend. My depression lifted. I suddenly broke through my block in playing the piano and was able to play the way I had always played. It was just amazing the freedom that I got from my decision to get out of Topeka. So I started looking around.

When I did my internship at Ohio State, I worked with another resident who subsequently went to New York where he became very successful in academic circles. He encouraged to me to come to New York to do my residency there. After my residency interview, he took me to a certain men's room at a certain subway station where there were twenty-five to thirty men having sex. The last one in line would remain in the entry hall and would warn everyone if anyone came in who was not suitable, so that everybody could suddenly go about whatever they were supposed to be doing until that person left and they could return to having sex. My colleague thought that the scene would turn me on to New York. However, it scared the hell out of me. It was too big, too expensive, and too free for me.

I ended up coming to Philadelphia. I didn't want to be in Washington—it was too southern for me; Boston was too cold; New York was too fast; but Philadelphia fit. So I came to the University of Pennsylvania in July 1964 as a third-year resident in my outpatient year. I established a connection with several good people who were residents at the time and who have gone on to develop stellar careers. After I had been there about three months, the chair of the department came back from sabbatical. He found himself with a fat resident who embarrassed him in a couple of conferences by knowing more about some things than he did. I began to get the impression that he was kind of gunning for me.

With that dynamic in the background, I got a telephone call from a couple in the King of Prussia area of Pennsylvania who told me that I was their cousin and asked me to come and visit. So during that summer I spent several afternoons with the couple. I took their oldest son (who was getting ready to leave for college) to dinner. During the course of that dinner, he asked me why I was not married. I told him that I was gay. He got very scared and went home and told his mother and father that I was gay. His father was an old military colleague of my department chairman and quickly let the chairman know what I had said. I then was called into the chairman's office and told, "You can either resign or I'll fire you." When I said, "What for?" he said, "For being homosexual and not telling us." I asked him what he would have done if I [had] told him. He said that he would not have taken me in the program. I gathered that he was under some pressure from his military buddy to do something about the matter, and that if he didn't do something about it, his buddy was going to go stir things up with the administration at Penn. I got a lawyer and was told that I should sue. However, I did not want to go back to the residency and I really didn't want any money from them. Penn did agree to give me a severance salary for six months. To my knowledge, all that was recorded at Penn was that I resigned and not for any reason.

Fortunately, I felt the need for therapy by that time. In Philadelphia there was the Association for Psychoanalysis and the Society for Psychoanalysis. The "association" was conservative and the "society" was liberal. The society had such people as Spurgeon English (who was the chair at Temple), John Benson, and Leon Saul. I asked for a recommendation from Leon Saul and was referred to Silas Warner. I was in analysis with him for four years and, from some of the interventions he made, I inferred that he would have liked for me to be straight. But, he never really came out and said that and seemed accepting of my being gay. But he did tell me that I should not even consider becoming a psychoanalyst because I was gay.

From September 1964 until January 1965 I lived off the six months severance pay from the University of Pennsylvania. I went to work at the Library of the College of Physicians of Philadelphia and wrote abstracts. My analyst said to me, "Are you still going to be a psychiatrist?" I lamented, "No one will take me." However, through some of my contacts, I met the superintendent of Norristown State Hospital, Carmela deRivas. I had a sense that this state-run psychiatric hospital in the northern suburbs of Philadelphia might take me. She talked with Penn and negotiated an agreement to have me work on Norristown's Med-Surgical Unit between February 1965 until July 1965 when I entered the next class.

After I entered the residency program, I realized that the residency director did not want me there. But Carmela supported me. They gave me the worst assignments. I was assigned to Building 11 as the only psychiatrist for 400 male patients. I also was assigned to Building 13, which was for the chronically incontinent patients. The protocol of the hospital before I got there was that if any male patient was incontinent in the rest of the hospital, he was assigned to Building 13. When the staff would take all the patients into the lunchroom, other staff would hose down the dayroom, and then, when the patients got through with lunch, they would hose down the dining room. And then they would hose down the bedrooms. They would hose down the rooms with high-pressure hoses four or five times a day. So I said to Carmela, "You want me to fix this?" And she said, "Do you think you can?" Essentially I set up a behavioral program rewarding patients who controlled their incontinence by sending them to state-run domiciles in the Pocono Mountains. I also told the other units that they could not send their incontinent patients to Building 13 anymore. When I left there, the building had almost no incontinent patients. So Carmela protected me from the residency director. Gradually, I felt as though it was all right to be out and I could be a psychiatrist and be gay. To this day, I still see members of the staff at Norristown State and I am very fond of the people there.

I finished my residency there in 1967 and, by that time, had started going down to Temple University Medical School to work in the first community mental health center based in the black ghetto of North Philadelphia. The chairman was Bruce Sloane, the director of the program was Al Gardner, and the Chief of the emergency section was Tony Panzetta. Now you have to understand that there were 300 people on the staff of the center. The period between 1967 and 1970 was the heyday of the community mental health center at Temple.

I also became active with the Health Care and Human Values Task Force. That task force was awarded $5,000 to study the professional response to death and dying. I used the money to create a local group in Philadelphia, called *Ars Moriendi,* which developed a membership of several hundred. I'll digress a moment. In 1974, *Ars Moriendi* received $75,000 to bring to Columbia, Maryland, all of the then-leaders in the field of death and dying—Elisabeth Kübler-Ross, Dame Cicely Saunders, Colin Murray Parkes, Herman Feifel, Robert Jay Lifton, Edwin Shneidman—and about seventy others for a five-day open discussion about issues in death, dying, and bereavement. This group became the International Work Group on Death, Dying and Bereavement, of which I was chair until 1979. That group continues to be active to this day.

Returning to my story, after my residency, I was pretty well-known by everyone at that point as being gay. I became part of [what we called] the Gay-P-A, a loose underground network of closeted gay psychiatrists who regularly attended the annual meetings of the American Psychiatric Association. In 1970, at the APA meeting in San Francisco, all of us watched Barbara Gittings (a Philadelphia activist who headed the gay component of the American Library Association) and Frank Kameny, PhD (an acerbic Harvard-trained astronomer from Washington, DC) picketing the APA. We in the Gay-P-A commented, "Isn't that nice," but we weren't about to do anything that might expose us.

So what happened back there in 1972? After [she crashed] the APA's Convocation of Fellows in Washington, DC, in 1970, the APA asked Barbara Gittings to be part of the panel "Lifestyles of Non-Patient Homosexuals." Barbara's lover, Kay Lahusen, noted that the panel had gays who were not psychiatrists and psychiatrists who were not gay. She said, "What we really need is a psychiatrist who is gay." Barbara decided to get letters from several gay psychiatrists, which were to be read without their names.

In the summer of 1970, my father died, which focused me on my death and dying work at that time. In that process I developed a friendship with a man with whom I later got involved intimately. In November 1971, I visited his home in New Hampshire when Barbara Gittings called and said, "John, we need you to be on a panel [in May 1972]," and I said, "Tell me about it." She said, "It's going to be a panel about homosexuality, and we need a gay psychiatrist." I said, "Sooo . . . ?!" She responded, "Well, look, you . . . um . . . think about it." She said that the Maurice Falk Foundation out of Pittsburgh had provided a grant to pay the travel expenses of a psychiatrist to be on a panel with Barbara Gittings, Judd Marmor, Robert Seidenberg, and a psychiatrist from Shepherd Pratt Psychiatric Hospital, Kent Robinson. They wanted someone on the panel who was gay.

In 1971 I was not feeling very secure. I was not [employed] full-time anywhere. I was only on the clinical faculty at Temple and did not have tenure. But I thought about it and realized it was something that had to be done. I had been thrown out of a residency because I was gay; I had lost a job because I was gay. That perspective needed to be heard from a gay psychiatrist by an audience that perhaps might be more inclined to listen to a psychiatrist. I told Barbara that I would participate on the panel but I could not do it as me. I didn't feel secure enough. Barbara asked what had to be done so that I could be on the committee. She then agreed to help me with a disguise.

Now, when you're my size, coming up with a disguise is not always easy. Fortunately, my lover at that time was a drama major and, with his assistance, we created an outfit. I wore this formal outfit that was several sizes too big with a blue shirt, and I had a rubber mask that went over my head that had different features from my own. My lover instructed me on how to make the mask look even more different.

The night that I was on the panel, my voice was disguised. Nobody knew who I was; the people for whom I worked didn't know it was I. So basically, my cover was clean. What actually I said was quite short:

Thank you, Dr. Robinson. I am a homosexual. I am a psychiatrist. I, like most of you in this room, am a member of the APA and am proud to be a member. However, tonight I am, insofar as it is possible, a "we." I attempt tonight to speak for many of my fellow gay members of the APA as well as for myself. When we gather at these conventions, we have a group, which we have glibly come to call the Gay-P-A. And several of us feel that it is time that real flesh and blood stand up before you and ask to be listened to and understood insofar as that is possible. I am disguised tonight in order that I might speak freely without conjuring up too much regard on your part about the particular WHO I happen to be. I do that mostly for your protection. I can assure you that I could be any one of more than a hundred psychiatrists registered at this convention. And the curious among you should cease attempting to figure out who I am and listen to what I say.

We homosexual psychiatrists must persistently deal with a variety of what we shall call "Nigger Syndromes." We shall describe some of them and how they make us feel.

As psychiatrists who are homosexual, we must know our place and what we must do to be successful. If our goal is academic appointment, a level of earning capacity equal to our fellows, or admission to a psychoanalytic institute, we must make certain that no one in a position of power is aware of our sexual orientation or gender identity. Much like the black man with the light skin who chooses to live as a white man, we cannot be seen with our real friends—our real homosexual family—lest our secret be known and our dooms sealed. There are practicing psychoanalysts among us who have completed their training analysis without mentioning their homosexuality to their analysts. Those who are willing to speak up openly will do so only if they have nothing to lose, then they won't be listened to.

As psychiatrists who are homosexuals, we must look carefully at the power which lies in our hands to define the health of others around us. In particular, we should have clearly in our minds our own particular understanding of what it is to be a healthy homosexual in a world which sees that appellation as an impossible oxymoron. One cannot be healthy and be homosexual, they say. One result of being psychiatrists who are homosexual is that we are required to be more healthy than our heterosexual counterparts. We have to make some sort of attempt through therapy or analysis to work problems out. Many of us who make that effort are still left with a sense of failure and of persistence of "the problem." Just as the black man must be superperson, so must we, in order to face those among our colleagues who know we are gay. We could continue to cite examples of this sort of situation for the remainder of the night. It would be useful, however, if we could now look at the reverse.

What is it like to be a homosexual who is also a psychiatrist? Most of us Gay-P-A members do not wear our badges into the Bayou Landing [a gay bar in Dallas] or the local Canal Baths. If we did, we could risk the derision of all the nonpsychiatrist homosexuals. There is much negative feeling in the homosexual community toward psychiatrists. And those of us who are visible are the easiest targets [on] which the angry can vent their wrath. Beyond that, in our own hometowns, the chances are that in any gathering of homosexuals, there is likely to be any number of patients or paraprofessional employees who might try to hurt us professionally in a larger community if those communities enable them to hurt us that way.

Finally, as homosexual psychiatrists, we seem to present a unique ability to marry ourselves to institutions rather than wives or lovers. Many of us work twenty hours daily to protect institutions that would literally chew us up and spit us out if they knew the truth. These are our feelings, and like any set of feelings, they have value insofar as they move us toward concrete action.

Here, I will speak primarily to the other members of the Gay-P-A who are present, not in costume tonight. Perhaps you can help your fellow psychiatrist friends understand what I am saying. When you are with professionals, fellow professionals, fellow psychiatrists who are denigrating the "faggots" and the "queers," don't just stand back, but don't give up your careers either. Show a little creative ingenuity; make sure you let your associates know that they have a few issues that they have to think through again. When fellow homosexuals come to you for treatment, don't let your own problems get in your way, but develop creative ways to let the patient[s] know that they're all right. And teach them everything they need to know. Refer them to other sources of information with basic differences from your own so that the homosexual will be freely able to make his own choices.

Finally, pull up your courage by your bootstraps and discover ways in which you and homosexual psychiatrists can be closely involved in movements which attempt to change the attitudes of heterosexuals—and homosexuals—toward homosexuality. For all of us have something to lose. We may not be considered for that professorship. The analyst down the street may stop referring us his overflow. Our supervisor may ask us to take a leave of absence. We are taking an even bigger risk, however, not accepting fully our own humanity, with all of the lessons it has to teach all the other humans around us and ourselves. This is the greatest loss: our honest humanity. And that loss leads all those others around us to lose that little bit of their humanity as well. For, if they were truly comfortable with their own homosexuality, then they could be comfortable with ours. We must use our skills and wisdom to help them—and us—grow to be comfortable with that little piece of humanity called homosexuality.

After the panel, I did a local radio talk show and was on the air for two hours as many of the Gay-P-A listened to my voice-disguised broadcast from one of the gay bars. The next year in 1973, Robert Spitzer came to our Gay-P-A meetings. By that time we had forty or fifty members. Dr. Spitzer then was instrumental in helping to remove the pathological diagnosis for homosexuality from the *Diagnostic and Statistical Manual*. (Consequently, I felt very betrayed when he recently stated that in his opinion gays could become straight.)

The year after the Dr. H. Anonymous episode, I was on the staff at Friends Hospital, a psychiatric hospital in Philadelphia. Again, a medical student perceived me as getting too close to him and may have said I came on to him—I don't know. I never had sex with him. But the medical student went to the administration, which called me in and said (and I liked this comment), "If you were gay and not flamboyant we would keep you. If you were flamboyant and not gay we would keep you. But since you are both gay and flamboyant, we cannot keep you." I therefore was terminated. Parenthetically, the administrator who made the comment was on the front row when I was Dr. H. Anonymous. He never knew it was I.

I then returned to the faculty at Temple. Tony Panzetta, who was chair by then, was not able at first to find any money to cover my salary. In 1975 I had a grant come in from the NIAAA [National Institute on Alcohol Abuse and Alcoholism] to become a drug and alcohol career teacher. Tony knew that I was gay but I was not actually out to him. That period between 1974 and 1978, however, was a very tenuous time for me. I feared even going to the gay psychiatrists' meetings. However, in 1978, I got associate professorship and tenure. The Dr. H. Anonymous event probably was the central event in my career. I was able to be "out" a lot more in my career after that. In 1978 when I got tenure at Temple I felt much more secure.

In 1980 to 1981, I was invited by Dame Cicely Saunders to come to England to help restructure the Education Centre of St. Christopher's Hospice in London. For that year I was the Director of Studies and Honorary Lecturer in the London Hospital Department of Psychiatry. I then returned to my faculty position at Temple until my retirement in 2000.

Many years ago, I purchased a large Victorian home in Germantown (a Philadelphia neighborhood). One of the medical students, David Hartman, who was quite famous because he was blind, worked with me at Friends Hospital. When he got married in 1974, three of the medical students who came to the wedding needed someplace to live right away. Although I had planned to set the house up for such arrangements, I hadn't done so yet. However, because they needed someplace right away, we managed. Over the years I had approximately forty medical students, many of them women, living in my home.

I am honored that people want to know about the Dr. H. Anonymous episode. At this point in my life, I am less active in the American Psychiatric Association and the Association of Gay and Lesbian Psychiatrists. I played the organ since I was twelve. I was originally part of the Disciples of Christ but later became an Episcopalian. Lately, however, I have been uncomfortable with the direction that the Episcopal Church is going. I have gone up as far as I can go in the political hierarchy of the church. So I'm looking for a home. I have the goal in the next three years of going to Australia for a year and maybe even staying. I don't know that I will be able to do so. I have diabetes, which has given me a retinopathy and, because of my weight, is not as easily controlled with insulin anymore. In 1997 I was diagnosed with sarcoidosis, which affects my balance and leaves me with a low red blood cell count on top of only 30 percent capacity in my lungs. So I don't know if I will ever get to go to Australia. But I am trying to get my house fixed up to sell it so that I can go. The loves of my life are my two Dobermans, Rocket and Sierra. You must put that in the article. My dogs have always been the light of my life: Toppest between 1972 and 1982, Micah between 1982 and 1990, and Zach between 1990 and 1997.

Dénouement

John E. Fryer, Dr. H. Anonymous, whose flamboyance and compulsion to test all the limits in his life, played a pivotal role in moving psychiatrists away from the concept of homosexuality as disease to the current, widely held belief that homosexuality is an essential characteristic of individuals which is independent of mental pathology. His gay professional contemporaries—more conservative, staid, traditional—could not, and did not, take the risks that Dr. Fryer took. Although the entire gay and lesbian community has benefited from Dr. Fryer's actions, it is his lesbian and gay professional contemporaries who have benefited most. From the Stonewall riots by transgendered and transvestite peoples, gay activism is replete with individuals who have been outside the traditional molds but who have been willing to risk scorn in the name of forging a place of acceptance in society. These are the heroes. This is John Fryer.

Chapter 2

An Interview with Charles Silverstein, PhD

Albert J. Sbordone

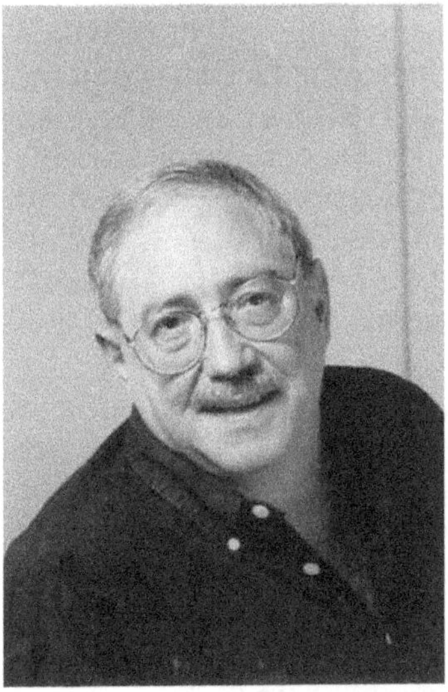

Introduction

I ring the bell and Charles greets me, his bulky frame comfortably clad in a plaid shirt whose tails hang out over khaki pants. He leads the way down a forty-foot hall which passes by his office on one side and a waiting room on the other. Sculptures, posters, drawings, and paintings invite pause and inquiry on the journey to the rest of his similarly decorated apartment.

My relationship with Charles Silverstein dates back almost twenty years. After our supervisory relationship ended, we gradually developed a close personal friendship. He excels at both. I know him as a gentle lion. He is a kind, generous, honest, and supportive friend. He is also a ferocious defender of scientific thinking and fairness. As we sit at his dining room table, readying ourselves to begin this interview, I am aware of

This chapter appeared originally under the same title in *Journal of Gay & Lesbian Psychotherapy* 7(4):49-61. Copyright 2003 The Haworth Press, Inc.

American Psychiatry and Homosexuality: An Oral History
Published by The Haworth Press, Inc., 2007. All rights reserved.
doi:10.1300/6049_03

the paternal transference that I and many others feel at times in his presence. I want this to go well. I want the reader to get to know the man behind the professional icon.

The public profile goes like this. On February 8, 1973, the Nomenclature Committee of the American Psychiatric Association (APA) convened to consider the issue of homosexuality. Should it be retained in or withdrawn from the *Diagnostic and Statistical Manual of Mental Disorders* (DSM)? At that meeting, Charles Silverstein, while still completing his doctoral dissertation in psychology, presented a powerful argument in favor of its withdrawal. By the end of that year, with a recommendation from that committee, the APA voted to drop homosexuality from the nomenclature.[1] The result of that action has had repercussions to this day in the fields of medicine, religion, and law.

At around the same time, Charles was engaged in other activities which would have a lasting impact upon the gay and lesbian community. In 1971, he was a cofounder of Identity House, a gay and lesbian peer counseling center in New York City. He later cofounded the Institute for Human Identity, a center for professional psychotherapy and training for gays and lesbians in New York City, in 1973. And, in 1975, he became the founding editor of the *Journal of Homosexuality.* All of these have endured and continue to serve the gay and lesbian community to this day.

By 1977, Charles had published one of the most important and widely read books in the gay community, *The Joy of Gay Sex*. He later appeared in a Canadian court to testify against that country's attempt to ban the book from crossing its borders. In that same year he published *A Family Matter: A Parent's Guide to Homosexuality.* In 1981, *Man to Man: Gay Couples in America* was on the bookshelves.

These are a smattering of Charles Silverstein's accomplishments. The question remains: "Who is the man behind them?"

JGLP: What was it like for you to train as a psychologist and to come out as a gay man in the late 1960s and early 1970s?

DR. SILVERSTEIN: I started my training at City College and did not come out at that time. It was a clinical program, and I had not the slightest doubt that I would have been thrown out if they knew. Then I went to Rutgers University and finished my PhD there; however, I was not out there either. Again, I felt that there was no chance that I'd ever stay if I came out. They would have thrown me out. There was no one out in those days in a graduate program in psychology.

And since I was living in the city, and going to school in New Brunswick, New Jersey, I could separate those two parts of my life. I came out here in Manhattan, with the Gay Activists Alliance [GAA], and continued my training in Rutgers.

It was certainly a split in my life, but one that I thought made great sense. All the medical students and psychiatric residents were doing exactly the same thing. As a gay liberationist, I needed that PhD because it gave me credibility. And I wasn't going to jeopardize getting it. So I was in the closet.

JGLP: What got you involved with GAA?

DR. SILVERSTEIN: I had finally come to terms with my homosexuality by having sex with a guy. The story of that event is published in *Boys Like Us*. And it was at that time that I realized how my repression of my homosexuality was such a harmful thing. I made a promise to myself to do something. And I heard about the Gay Activists Alliance.

The first time I went down, I parked my car far away from the building. I saw this line of guys outside, waiting to get into a dance which they held every Saturday night. And I was so terrified. They all seemed to be having so much fun enjoying each other and touching each other. I just turned around and got back into my car and drove away really quickly.

But the first step had been taken, and within a week I went back to one of their meetings. And so, associating myself with this organization, I could not only do something for gay civil rights, but for myself. I became very active with them. I've always been a very political person, and so it was natural. And it was there that I met my lover, William.

JGLP: A lot of your earliest work critiqued the diagnosis of homosexuality as nothing more than a means of social control that kept gay men feeling ashamed, in a state of low self-esteem, and often depressed. In this state, many gay men sought the help of therapists, to try to become heterosexual. Your work in this area has been so very impassioned. Did you, yourself, have such an experience?

DR. SILVERSTEIN: Oh sure. The first time I went to see a therapist I was sixteen. I was madly in love with a close friend, madly in love with him. He was absolutely wonderful. And, of course, I wanted to touch him all over, but I couldn't. I was terrified of these feelings.

So, I went to a family physician, and I told him that I had homosexual tendencies. That was the term of the day, "homosexual tendencies." So he wrote Kings County Mental Health Clinic, and he got rid of me just as soon as he possibly could.

I was under the impression that my meeting with someone there would be confidential. I was led into this office, with a man sitting behind a desk, smoking a cigar. And in the corner were two other guys with pads, writing down everything I said. So here I was, hoping it would be confidential, and there were three people in the room.

I talked for a while. I asked him questions, and then he led me down the hall to another person's office. I guess he was a psychiatrist. I walked in there along with the first three people, and the psychiatrist was in there with another person. So, there I was in a room with five people. And, the psychiatrist had a Fu Manchu mustache. He seemed very strange to me. I just said to him: I'm getting out of here. And I did.

When I was in college, I went to see someone in Kingston, New York. And, after I came out of college, and I was teaching, I went into psychoanalysis. Over the course of eight more years, I saw two different analysts.

When I walked into the office of the first analyst, I told him that I wanted to be cured. I said to him, "If you won't undertake that, then I don't want to see you." In those days, professionals wrote that sometimes homosexuals could not be cured. Sometimes, because they are so far gone, it is better to adjust them to their homosexuality. And I did not want to be adjusted. If he had said to me that he thought it would be better for me to be adjusted, I would have walked out of his office, too. I was very much the kind of person who had this low self-esteem, depression, and feelings of shame that I wrote about later.

JGLP: What was your motivation? Why were you so determined that you were going to change? What made you want to be straight?

DR. SILVERSTEIN: You know, it's all the cliché answers: the shame it would represent in the family; the feeling of being a pervert; being a criminal; losing all my friends; not being able to get married and have children. And, I was isolated. I didn't know anyone else who was gay. How would I know them? They were all in the closet the same as I was, except for those who were drag queens here in New York.

JGLP: You mentioned the shame this would bring on your family. What was your family like?

DR. SILVERSTEIN: Well, my brother was six and a half years older, and was my father's favorite son. I wasn't very close to my father. I was closer to my mother. There's no question I was her favorite son.

Ours was very much the standard relationship you'd have in that generation between a Jewish mother and her son. The Jewish mother did not know that there was a physical or psychological difference between her and her children. The very idea would be rejected as unfathomable. Anytime the Jewish son did something that she didn't like, it was like you had literally ripped flesh from her body. So it was very important to be good. And I was good most of the time. I mean, to her I was very bad much of the time, but bad only meant not listening to your mother. You didn't pick up your socks. You didn't listen to your teacher. But these took on incredible importance. This is a standard story. There's nothing unique about this. You get this from any person who's Jewish from that generation, gay or straight.

I once, some years ago, saw three patients one evening, all of whom were Jewish. Each one came in complaining about his mother. Each one was screaming, and hollering, and cursing, and yelling. At the end of the evening, not only could I not tell the difference between their mothers, I could not tell the difference between their mothers and my mother. That's where I came to my theory that there was only one Jewish mother in the whole world running from house to house to do all these things. This is why she is complaining how tired she is, and how much work she has to do. It was all very much the same. But I was convinced I had to be good.

Later on in life, I learned what an advantage it would have been if I [had been] a bad kid and [had] played with the other bad kids. Because they had a much freer life than I did. Of course, if my mother told my father that I'd been bad, he'd come in and take off his belt and whack my ass with it, and smack me.

He worked at night, including weekends, and slept during the day. His days off were during the week. He was sleeping when we were up, and when we were sleeping he was working. So we never saw him very much. We hardly knew he lived in the house. He would bring home money. On Sundays, he would generally come home with bagels and lox. But we just didn't know him. He was also a man with a temper, and not much patience. So he would bat the hell out of us from time to time.

It was only later on in life, as a very late teenager, that I got to know him at all—and that's because he had a heart attack. When he went back to work, the doctor didn't want him to throw the bundles of newspapers into the truck, so I would go and help him. That is where I saw him in a totally different context. At work, he was actually very warm and friendly. He had lots of friends there, and they joked with each other.

You know, through osmosis, you identify with parents, and you take on behaviors that you are not aware of until much later in life. I think that, unquestionably, I learned that how my mother treated my father, her husband, was the model of how you treat a man. If he was sleeping much of the time, he was a sleeping volcano. She learned not to disturb the volcano, because he would get violent. Now, I don't want to overdo that. It's not as if he were beating everybody up. But he used to beat me and my brother for misbehaving. What he defined as misbehaving. I never saw him hit my mother. She learned how to quiet him, to keep his anger down. That's what I learned, and I think that is what I did with men through[out] my life: not disturbing the volcanoes that might be in them, anticipating their needs, and taking care of them as my mother took care of my father.

JGLP: In "Siren's Song," your chapter in *Boys Like Us,* you said that you had thought that your parents were at the root of your homophobia. In what way do you think that is true or not true today?

DR. SILVERSTEIN: I still think the major problem people have in coming out is shame because it would be a shame in the family, a potential rejection. It is a very isolating experience. In my day, there were lots of children who were literally, that very night they came out, thrown out of the house and told not to come back. I don't think that happens very much today—but, still, it's a matter of great shame.

How does the message of shame get through so powerfully? I'm not sure what is the answer. It's not as if they talked about homosexuals in my house.

The schoolyard probably had something to do with it. There is an association between masculinity, and the lack of it, and homosexuality and heterosexuality. So that the gay boy who is not very good at sports is identified as a sissy, which he probably is. Most often he gets the gay position, right field, or left out. I suspect that the reason is more about issues of masculinity than issues of sexual orientation. It's about being a real boy.

I had an advantage. Even though I wasn't good in sports, I was big and strong. So if someone teased me, I could wallop him. This is the only lesson I learned from my father. I'll tell you a story. I was in junior high, and there was one guy there who was picking on me. You know, he was taller and bigger and stronger. I can't remember why he was picking on me, probably because I was standing in the same place for fifteen seconds. He was just a bully.

So I went home and complained to my parents. They were very upset. My mother, being a mother, said, "You have to stay away from him." Now, there could be nothing more absurd. My father understood that avoiding him wouldn't work, and he said to me, "You have to fight him." This I thought a profoundly stupid idea, and I said that this boy would beat the hell out of me. And my father said, "It doesn't make any difference. The important thing is to hit him. If you do that, even though he beats you up, you will have made the point. He will not touch you again. He'll go after someone else."

I went to school the next day, and this guy came over to me and hit me. So I walloped him back. Then he proceeded to beat the shit out of me, with the usual big crowd of kids watching. Some of them thought that I was the stupidest person in the world. I had a bloody nose, and my shirt was ripped, but *he* had a bloody nose, and *his* shirt was ripped.

In this, the only advice my father ever gave to me, he was right. You have to stand up to the bully. That is an experience I have never forgotten: that you can't let the bully get away with it. You gotta wallop him, good and hard.

I think, in many ways, this was the metaphor for my attitude about gay liberation. That I am not gonna be cowered by the bullies out there, whether it is society, the law, religion, or the psychiatric profession. I'm going to go out, and I'm going to wallop the bastards in the face. I'm pretty proud that I did that.

JGLP: It wasn't long after you came out that you became a dynamic and visionary leader in the gay psychology movement. Of which accomplishment are you most proud?

DR. SILVERSTEIN: Oh, that's easy. It was my work to delete homosexuality as a mental disorder from the *Diagnostic and Statistical Manual* of the American Psychiatric Association. That was clearly the single most important thing that was accomplished by the gay liberation movement because the psychiatric profession has so much status in our society.

We were convinced that having homosexuality deleted from the nomenclature would have a profound effect on our survival. But, we were attacking something more important than the diagnosis of homosexuality. We were attacking the use of moral beliefs as the foundation for declaring a person mentally well or ill. However, that's an issue with which we were only partially successful.

JGLP: Looking back on that moment, thirty years ago, when you were delivering your testimony to the Nomenclature Committee of the APA, can you recall what it was that you were feeling?

DR. SILVERSTEIN: A sense of being completely right, and that I was going to win. But I would say that it was not just me. There were, I think, five of us there, and I think every one of those people would answer the same way today. And, perhaps I was feeling self-righteousness, a trait of which I have a decent amount.

I was sitting in front of this committee, having composed this document of which I was very proud. In addition, exactly a week earlier, my lover William had moved in with me. So I was very happy about that. Just sitting in front of the committee and reading my paper, I knew that we were going to win this battle. It was merely a matter of waiting till they came around to our side. That's what I thought, and without the slightest ambivalence on my part. I knew that what I had written was very clever and very competent.

And they were very impressed. They were expecting a gay-liberation diatribe, and I knew they were expecting that. So I thought that it made more sense to play in their ballpark, the ballpark of diagnosis. In preparation for that, I had spent a couple of months doing nothing but reading about diagnoses since the time of the ancient Greeks. I came to understand the nature of diagnosis.

I wrote the paper the night before the presentation on my little typewriter. I walked in the next day knowing that I had done the right thing. I think some of them were actually amused, which is a perfectly reasonable response to a listing of diagnoses over the ages—syphilophobia, pathologic mendacity, masturbation. You know, masturbation had been a mental illness since 1942, and it is still considered a mental illness by some of our colleagues.

I threw back at them their diagnoses over the decades, and how funny it all sounds now, and pointed out that their fun had hurt a lot of people. I ended by saying to them, "Don't do it anymore."

JGLP: Did you have any idea at that time of the enormous impact your words would have on the lives of countless gay men and lesbians, then and in the future?

DR. SILVERSTEIN: I think we did. We couldn't know how many caucuses in professional organizations would be arranged, how many gay liberation groups in colleges. But we knew that the two most important things that had happened were that they could no longer use homosexuality as a mental illness in promulgating laws against gay people, and that it would give lawyers the opportunity of challenging the sodomy laws. We understood those things. Now, whether we knew exactly how far that would go, I don't know. But I think we were really very cognizant of what we were doing.

JGLP: Did your Jewish heritage have anything to do with your fight against what you have referred to as "sexual ethnic cleansing"?

DR. SILVERSTEIN: Oh, absolutely. There was a lot of talk in my family, in my extended family, about discrimination against Jews. Some of my uncles were socialists, and a couple of them were Communists in the early days. When they found out what Russia was really like, they stopped. But there were a lot of Jews who were socialists in those days—in my parent's generation—who were members of the socialist organization. Their concern was the treatment of Jews in America. They were also the people that started all these black organizations: the Urban League, the NAACP [National Association for the Advancement of Colored People]. They were all started by Jews.

I think that instilled in me a sense of fair play that affected me deeply, and it certainly did have a lot to do with my choices in life about battling against my society. In that way, I was very much like my family.

JGLP: What affected your choice in art?

DR. SILVERSTEIN: I've become interested in art that represents the manner in which people have suffered. For instance, that's my race-music wall—a bunch of song sheets that people used to use at one time when there was no radio or television. They would sit around and sing with the piano. All of them represent stereotypes of black people that were common in those days.

There's a picture out front of four Vietcong soldiers reading mail from home. I was the leader of the strike in New Jersey against the Vietnam War, so I wanted to get that picture.

The latest picture is done by an artist by the name of Van Nath who was in Phnom Penh during the period of Pol Pot and the Khmer Rouge. There were tens of thousands of people who went into a prison in Phnom Penh, Toul Sleng, and only seven survived—he was one of them. The reason he survived was because he was an artist, so he could paint portraits of Pol Pot. They kept him alive for that reason. The Pol Pot regime was supported by the United States government. The great shame of all of this is that we virtually encouraged Pol Pot to kill somewhere between one and two million of his people. But, Van Nath painted a number of paintings of his experiences in prison. So for over a year now I've been trying to get a painting of his.

So, much of my interest in folk art is as a reminder of how cruel people can be to others.

JGLP: Throughout most all of your public life, you were also in a relationship with your partner, William Bory. This was a relationship that lasted over twenty years until he sadly died of AIDS in 1993. Tell me about that relationship.

DR. SILVERSTEIN: I would say that I loved William at first sight. I loved him even more the night he died. It was the intervening twenty years that were the problem. William had many attributes I did not have. He was intellectually brilliant. He was beautiful. He was self-educated and cultured in a way that I have never been. His immense knowledge was very interesting to me. He knew everything about ancient civilizations. And, he was very hot in bed.

Going back to what I said earlier, I treated him very much the way my mother treated my father. That is, to anticipate his needs; to provide for them, which is deadly; and to calm the volcano that was in him. There were times we had that were absolutely wonderful. Most of the trips we went on were fabulous. When we'd go on trips, I was very good about planning where we would go, the itinerary, and the hotels. He would sit down for the next month and read about the country, the history, the archaeology, the places to go—he would know them cold. When we went to Rome, he said he wanted to get married in the atrium of the vestal virgins. He knew exactly where the vestal virgins' atrium was because he read a guide to Rome that was written 2,000 years ago. When we went to Egypt he taught himself hieroglyphics. So, he knew things that no tour guide would know, and he would tell me about them—as long as there weren't other people around. If other people were around, he would walk out.

JGLP: Was William interested in the issues that you were addressing in your work?

DR. SILVERSTEIN: Oh, absolutely. He thought that what I was doing was very important. He was very proud of what I was doing. That represented real masculinity to him. He was a firm supporter, though occasionally he would try to trip me up. I was once speaking at a conference at the University of Pennsylvania, and he was in the back of the room while I was speaking. He was exposing himself, trying to get me to laugh. But he did it in a way that other people couldn't see it, except me. That would be the sort of thing he would do.

We had fun, traveling, fighting with other people. We certainly shared moral values and had very similar senses of humor. He was very much an ally. All this is about passion. We shared that passion. And the passion wasn't necessarily about sex. We had sex, but that's not what it was about. It was about representing something, fighting for something. And criticizing other people. He was very good at that.

JGLP: How did his death affect you?

DR. SILVERSTEIN: Oh, God! Relief, sorrow. As you know, he had been quite sick and had made some very bad decisions about what he was going to do. First becoming alcoholic, then becoming a crack addict—that was a big strain on me. Of course, just taking care of someone who was dying of AIDS is a strain. So the night he died, I felt a great sense of relief.

What subsequently happened is that, as the years have gone on and on, I have remembered the good times much more than I've remembered the bad times. I no longer talk to him. He's sitting over there, on the bookshelf, with his beret on the ashes, and I mainly remember the good times. Of which there were many.

JGLP: Did anything change in your relationships with patients during his illness and after his death?

DR. SILVERSTEIN: Well, one's relationships with patients are very complicated. While William was ill, I was running support groups for people treating AIDS patients. In addition, I had a private practice, where there were a number of people who were HIV positive and who had AIDS and were dying. I was surrounded by all of this, and taking care of other people who were involved with illness and dying. I can remember at some of the support groups I conducted, saying to myself, "I wish they would shut up. I've heard enough, and I wish they would talk about something else." Because, you know, it was just all around me. People coming out today cannot understand that period when everybody was dying because things are so different now. I wanted them to shut up, occasionally. They never did, and I didn't tell them to, of course. But it certainly affected me that way. So when William died, a large part of the stress was taken off me, and I found I could listen to the needs of patients better than I could before.

JGLP: In a life so full of accomplishments, what have you not done that you'd like to do?

DR. SILVERSTEIN: There is never an end to my desire to travel. I always thought I was born at least a century too late—that I would have wanted to have been born the second son of a British duke. I say the second son because that was the time when they had primogeniture. The first son inherits the title and all the responsibilities. The second son gets a stipend and has nothing to do whatsoever—and they'd just as soon he not even be in the house. So if I were the second son, I would have all of this money supplied to me on a yearly basis, for which I wouldn't have to do a stitch of work, and I could go traveling. I would spend six months of each year planning the travel of the next six months. That would have been heaven for me. See, I'm planning a trip right now. I haven't seen the whole world yet.

JGLP: What about professionally?

DR. SILVERSTEIN: Well, this is going to get me into enormous trouble. One of the things that nomenclature change has proven in the last thirty years is that gay professionals can be just as fascist in their positions as straight professionals. I want to fight against that. I want to begin speaking out against our colleagues who condemn other gay people's sexual behavior. I'm thinking of all of the people who are diagnosed as having one kind of sexual perversion or another, for no other reason than it's not statistically normal, and that it is a violation of social mores. I'm thinking of anyone involved in S&M, whether you're a top or a bottom; people who are into drag; people who are into fetishes. Lots of our gay professional colleagues look down upon these.

For example, many of our colleagues diagnose sexual compulsion. The issue is that anyone who jerks off more than I do is suffering from a sexual compulsion or addiction. They never distinguish between those two—they don't know the difference.

What we were doing in 1973 was attacking the idea that you have the right to diagnose these people as suffering from some illness because you've identified with society's rules; that it's not good to suck toes, for instance. The unfortunate thing is that, right now, a lot of our gay colleagues are doing the same thing. So they've turned out to be just as oppressive as the heterosexual professionals who preceded them. I want to do what I can to attack that point of view. I want to bring a sense of morality about diagnosis back into the nomenclature, by dropping morality as its prerequisite.

Also, many of our colleagues today attack the idea that we can cure homosexuals. Whether we can change the sexual orientation of homosexuals is irrelevant; it is immoral to attempt to do so. Sexuality is like a flower—it unfolds—and it is very much a part of us. The attempt to change that is immoral, whether there is a technique that can change it or not. You don't have a right to make that attempt. Now, that is a moral position.

Finally, there are a couple of books I want to write. I'm trying to get my latest book published right now. It's called *For the Ferryman*. It's the story of my work in gay liberation and my life with William. A fabulous book.

JGLP: People have labeled you in different ways: a hero, a troublemaker, the grandfather of gay psychology. What would you call yourself, and why?

DR. SILVERSTEIN: I'm just a psychologist. It is true that I am impassioned about a lot of things. Of the many criticisms people have had of me, I don't think anyone has ever criticized me for being dull and uninteresting. I have friends in New Jersey who talk about this all the time. I have the capacity to walk into a room, anywhere, and everything starts getting upset and excited. And there's a certain amount of truth there. I don't swim downstream. I can't tell you exactly the reason why I don't swim downstream. But, I speak my mind. And I really like that.

NOTE

1. Editor's Note: For a fuller account of those events, see Bayer, R. (1981), *Homosexuality and American Psychiatry: The Politics of Diagnosis*. New York: Basic Books.

SELECTED BIBLIOGRAPHY

Books

Silverstein, C. & White, E. (1977), *The Joy of Gay Sex*. New York: Crown.

Silverstein, C. (1977), *A Family Matter: A Parent's Guide to Homosexuality*. New York: McGraw-Hill.

Silverstein, C. (1981), *Man to Man: Gay Couples in America*. New York: William Morrow.

Silverstein, C., ed. (1991), *Gays, Lesbians and Their Therapists: Studies in Psychotherapy*. New York: W. W. Norton.

Silverstein, C. & Picano, F. (1992), *The New Joy of Gay Sex*. New York: HarperCollins.

Silverstein, C. & Picano, F. (2003), *The Joy of Gay Sex*, Third Edition. New York: HarperCollins.

Book Chapters

Silverstein, C. (1991), Psychotherapy and medical treatment of homosexuality. In: *Homosexuality: Research Implications for Public Policy*, eds. J. Gonsiorek & J.A. Weinrich. Newbury Park, CA: Sage Publications, pp. 101-114.

Silverstein, C. (1991), Psychotherapy and psychotherapists: A history. In: *Gays, Lesbians and Their Therapists: Studies in Psychotherapy*, ed. C. Silverstein. New York: Norton, pp. 1-14.

Silverstein, C. (1991), When the therapist is more anxious than the patient. In: *Gays, Lesbians and Their Therapists: Studies in Psychotherapy,* ed. C. Silverstein. New York: Norton, pp. 240-252.

Silverstein, C. (1996), Siren's song. In: *Boys Like Us: Gay Writers Tell Their Coming-Out Stories,* ed. P. Merla. New York: Avon Books, pp. 115-123.

Silverstein, C. (1996), The medical treatment of homosexuality. In: *Textbook of Homosexuality and Mental Health,* eds. R. P. Cabaj & T. S. Stein. Washington, DC: American Psychiatric Press, pp. 3-16.

Silverstein, C. (1997), The origin of the gay psychotherapy movement. In: *A Queer World,* ed. M. Duberman. New York: New York University Press, pp. 358-381.

Papers

Silverstein, C. (1976-1977), Even psychiatry can profit from its past mistakes. *J. Homosexuality,* 2(2):153-158.

Silverstein, C. (1977), Symposium on homosexuality and the ethics of behavioral intervention (paper no. 2). *J. Homosexuality,* 2(3):205-211.

Silverstein, C. (1984), The ethical and moral implications of sexual classification: A commentary. *J. Homosexuality,* 9(4):29-38.

Silverstein, C. (2003), The religious conversion of homosexuals: Subject selection is the *voir dire* of psychological research. *J. Gay & Lesbian Psychotherapy,* 7(3): 31-53.

Chapter 3

An Interview with Lawrence Hartmann, MD

Jack Drescher

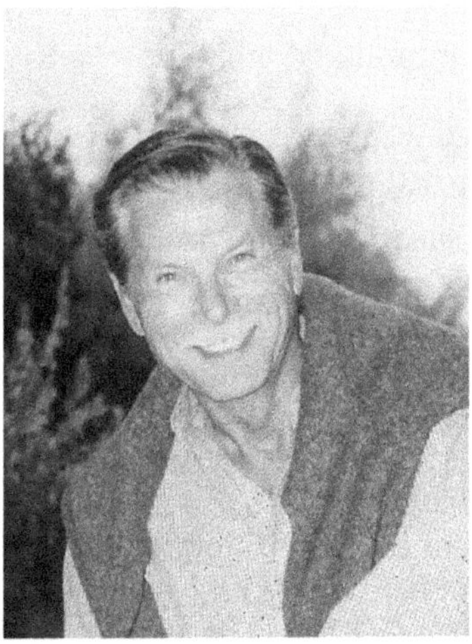

Lawrence Hartmann, the son of two psychoanalysts, grew up in New York City in the 1940s and 1950s. He went to Harvard College, to Oxford University as a Rhodes Scholar, and then to Harvard Medical School. Dr. Hartmann was an intern in Pediatrics at UC San Francisco, and went on to do his residency in adult psychiatry and a fellowship in child and adolescent psychiatry at Mass Mental Health Center/Harvard—while also being psychoanalyzed. Dr. Hartmann has taught at Harvard Medical School since then (in his own words as a "rather minor clinical professor of psychiatry").

Dr. Hartmann's interests in dynamic and social psychiatry, in biopsychosocial integration, in women, children, minorities, homosexuality, and human rights have led him to much activity and several leadership positions in both child and adult psychiatric organizations. This includes having served on or leading many committees and councils, helping to reform the American Psychiatric Association

This chapter appeared originally under the same title in *Journal of Gay & Lesbian Psychotherapy* 10(1):123-137.

American Psychiatry and Homosexuality: An Oral History
Published by The Haworth Press, Inc., 2007.
doi:10.1300/6049_04

(APA), and helping the APA to remove homosexuality from its diagnostic manual in 1973. After serving as Speaker of the APA Assembly and then Area Trustee and Vice President, Dr. Hartmann was President of the APA from 1991 to 1992. Since that time, he has remained a member of APA's Board of Trustees. He helped organize and took part in several psychiatry and human rights missions (Chile, South Africa, the former Soviet Union), and led a post–Iron Curtain Traveling University of Psychiatry to Poland, Czechoslovakia, and Hungary.

Dr. Hartman currently continues to teach at Harvard and has a two-thirds-time private practice in adult and child psychiatry in Cambridge.

JGLP: Tell us something about your background and what led you to become a psychiatrist.

DR. HARTMANN: I was born into a widely educated psychiatric and psychoanalytic family. My father was a well-known psychoanalyst, an analysand of Freud's, a theorist of ego psychology, and eventually a sort of dean of international psychoanalysis in the mid–twentieth century, when analysis was at its height.[1] My mother was a pediatrician who later became a psychiatrist and a child and adult psychoanalyst. I was born in Vienna, but my family moved to Paris when I was a year old, so I spoke French before anything else. We then moved to French-speaking Switzerland, and came to New York when I was about three and a half; I promptly forgot French and learned English, although I relearned French as a teenager.

I grew up in a world of interesting, cultured, cultivated upper-upper-middle-class New Yorkers—full of psychoanalysts, artists, and scientists. I was a rather happy child, and liked, admired, and respected my parents. My interest in child psychiatry certainly owes something to my mother. I loved school, and I was sent to excellent private schools all through my life, where I had creative teachers and a remarkable education, and had some trouble choosing among many and various thoughts as to what I might do with my life. I thought of becoming a writer, an actor, a playwright, a scientist, an English professor, a diplomat—something in government, and something to do with social issues and welfare and health issues. Eventually I decided that psychiatry combined humane, scientific, and artistic interests very well.

I liked my liberal arts college education at Harvard and studied, among other things, a lot of history and literature, before going on to Oxford for two years as a Rhodes Scholar, and earning two additional degrees, in English literature. At Harvard Medical School, I did not much enjoy the first two (regimented preclinical) years, but liked the next years when I began to work with patients. I went on to UC–San Francisco as a pediatric intern, and then came back to Harvard Medical School, to Mass Mental Health Center (MMHC),[2] which at that time was widely considered as probably the best place in the world to be trained in psychiatry.

It was a warm and lively and challenging place. There were lots of analysts and many basic scientists. Anybody good in Massachusetts in any field connected with psychiatry or analysis wanted to be attached to MMHC, and usually was. It had a remarkably large and stimulating residency program. Boston also felt like the right distance from New York, where I had grown up. Boston was separate and not my parents' city, but it was easy to get to New York, which I loved for theatre and opera and concerts and museums and all kinds of reasons. I liked going to see my parents and family friends, in the city or at my parents' weekend house. I liked living in Boston and then Cambridge, and I have lived here most of my life since college—with only a little time-out living in England and in California.

I am a very analytic psychiatrist, but clearly, like everyone else my age, I have also learned many things about social and biological and integrative psychiatry. I began looking for social psychiatric issues, and early on organized and helped with some interesting projects and minor crusades. As a resident, I discovered that Massachusetts' psychiatry residents were paid less than those in any other state of the union. This helped remarkably quickly in getting the state to pay us a bit more. I also learned that the four women in my residency class of twenty-five were being paid less than the men. The whole class agreed to ask the training director to pay us all equally, which was done. I got psychiatrists to volunteer to do work in prisons. It turned out I was fairly good at having a social conscience about issues and injustices, and at getting people to do things about them. That was well before I began doing public things that had direct relevance to gay and lesbian sexual issues.

JGLP: How do you think being gay affected your psychiatric career choices and your career development?

DR. HARTMANN: I think gradually accepting and being gay slowed me down in some ways, and stimulated me in others. Though I was in many ways an insider and part of the establishment, it made me face minority issues more fully. I had read, more than most of my peers, the rather awful "gayness is major pathology" psychoanalytic literature of the mid–twentieth century. I was discouraged and angered by that, and had qualms about the possibility of having to confront and fight the analytic establishment in order to go through analytic training in the late 1960s and early 1970s. I was analyzed (1965-1972), as most of us in leading psychiatric residencies then were, during residency and afterward, and my analysis taught me a good many useful things about myself and others. My analyst, who was a senior Freudian Boston-establishment training analyst, talked with me several times about what would happen if—an obvious-looking career path to take—I, as a bisexual or gay man, applied to the conservative (and at that time only) analytic institute in Boston. The American Psychoanalytic Association (APsaA) had never knowingly had an openly gay psychoanalyst. We (and others I asked) were not sure the APsaA had even ever had a gay person apply. I think I would have been unwilling (or unable?) to lie in my own training about such a large part of myself as sexuality, although I know that others have felt they had to, and I respect their pragmatic decision in doing that.

I think it was impossible at that time to be openly gay and to be a psychiatric resident in any good program in America—or, as far as I know, to be, in the 1960s, an excellent and respected bisexual or gay analytic psychiatrist. It was if anything even more impossible to be openly gay then and be a psychoanalytic candidate or analyst. It is hard for younger colleagues in 2004 fully to imagine or comprehend how very much of homosexuality was illegal and heavily disapproved of at that time. This area was a major obstacle in my life and in my self-respect. I was often unhappy, and sometimes in despair. I knew of no role models. I was unsure it could be done.

My analyst was aware that I was well-known, reasonably well-liked and respected, effective, trained and then teaching at a good program, and the son of one of the most famous and respected analysts around. The Boston institute, she thought, would have had a hard time saying no. Nevertheless, I rather thought they would have said no, and we both thought about that and its implications. Additionally, aside from the gayness issue, I thought that analytic training, at that point, in Boston, though excellent in some ways, seemed to me too rigid, obedient, and hierarchical—a bit too much like Jesuit training. I was and am very analytic—in addition to being analyzed I was supervised by about a dozen analysts, and have read and used a lot of analytic ideas and evidence and style—but I did not apply to the Boston Psychoanalytic Institute. I did some things in child psychiatry. I wrote a bit. I saw patients and began teaching and administering at Harvard. If I had chosen and been allowed to go into analytic training, I would probably have developed and done fewer public psychiatric things as quickly as I did.

In 1970, Cambodia and Kent State happened just prior to the APsaA and APA meetings, and that angered many of us, but also was very stimulating to those of us who thought that psychiatry ought to have a social conscience and do something about events and public policies that have psychiatric relevance. I think I had the political sense and sensitivity to make use of some of the turmoil of the late 1960s and early 1970s in directions that turned out to be useful toward the 1973 APA decision about homosexuality.

Though already a member, I felt an angry outsider in the APA in May 1970. It appalled me, and others, that the organization's leaders would not comment on, or even listen to its members about, Cambodia and Kent State. I decided to look at what the APA was, and what my local Northern New England (soon to become the Massachusetts) Psychiatric Society (NNEPS) was, and what I could do to inject social issues and values into the organizations' concerns. I joined the NNEPS Social Issues Committee, and I also began, with some others, to found and run a national group called the Committee for Concerned Psychiatrists (CFCP). This very quickly, in the early 1970s, nominated and got elected some very liberal and social-psychiatrically thoughtful people into the APA leadership—which was absolutely key to 1973. CFCP helped create a climate of real change in organized psychiatry, building partly on anti–Vietnam War energy, and partly on the major recent civil rights advances for blacks, as well as work for women's and children's issues.

Gay people were disparaged, left out, badly treated, and harmed by mid–twentieth century analysis and psychiatry. When I sought to help create a climate of change, where social issues would be included, I did not begin by doing that predominantly as a gay man pushing gay issues. In fact, I probably had more standing to work on gay issues because I was a young and fairly articulate establishment psychiatrist who had many connections and cared a lot about many social issues that were widely felt to be both right and neglected. To be forceful and direct about gay issues at the time, or even interested in gay issues, nearly immediately labeled you as probably gay yourself, and certainly scientifically and characterologically suspect. The few analysts who wrote about gay people tended to describe them as nasty psychopaths, close to psychosis. I am not making this up! Most leading psychiatrists and analysts, with a very few courageous exceptions like Judd Marmor, did not touch anything having to do with gay issues with any real objectivity, neutrality, or sympathy. "Gay psychiatrist" was not a category. I was not aware, in the late 1960s, that any existed. Some, it later turned out, had existed, but were closeted; and many of those tended to be relatively conservative socially and organizationally and, for quite a while, for many reasons, including fear, had not wanted or been able to push gay issues publicly.

JGLP: What was your role in the events leading up to, and culminating in, the 1973 APA decision to remove homosexuality from the DSM?

DR. HARTMANN: There were several things that I did, and I am very pleased to have been part of that 1973 decision. Many people were involved. It was not just science and not just politics. It was not just the APA Board. It was not just [Robert] Spitzer, or one APA committee; it was not just one or two or three outside groups. There was a climate of change and there were a lot of people who came together and did a lot of cooperative work, sometimes without talking to one another, sometimes aware of one another, sometimes not.

One of the things that I did was to create, with some others, a major change in what had been a guild-directed, conservative APA, shifting it into being an organization that looked for and embraced social psychiatric issues. The APA became markedly more active and helpful on black issues, women's issues, minority population issues, and gay issues. Some of the people that the CFCP got into positions of power were relatively socially liberal academics, from major cities and universities, rather than small-town, more purely money-and-guild-oriented psychiatrists. We had remarkable success in getting nominated and elected APA presidents, VPs, treasurers, and secretaries, for several years, including Al Friedman, Judd Marmor, John Spiegel, Jack Weinberg, and Viola Bernard. Each of them was extremely effective and contributed to new APA momentum and possibilities.

JGLP: It seems the APA was converted.

DR. HARTMANN: Changed, yes. In 1970 to 1973, specific gay issues percolated upward in and around the APA from several places. There were some demonstrations at APA meetings. There were closeted but useful Gay-P-A cocktail parties at APA meetings. There was a breakup of one scientific session where a behavioral therapist was promulgating coercive/aversive behavior therapy—then quite common—aimed at trying to stop gay people from being gay. There also was effective drama, as when the late John Fryer showed up in a mask to conceal his identity on an APA panel, where he spoke movingly as an anonymous gay psychiatrist.[3] There was a panel on gayness at the Hawaii APA meeting, where I think Marmor and Stoller spoke well, and also a smart nonpsychiatrist writer, Ron Gold, whose talk, urging the end of calling gayness an illness, was memorably titled "Stop It! You're Making Me Sick!" One thing I did was help create an activist APA climate in Washington, and I had the luck to help put in some specific people as leaders in the APA who were then very receptive and eager to do pro-gay things in 1973.

Vietnam War, women's and black issues, and then gay issues, helped fuel the idea that psychiatry had to be more creative about acknowledging and taking part in social issues that affected mental health and mental illness. We shifted the center of gravity away from a very conservative APA to far more progressive leadership, with new officers and a new medical director, whom we helped choose. (Even at our young age, the CFCP was consulted about and helped choose a liberal, decent, and creative medical director, Mel Sabshin.) There were also structural things with bylaws, the board of trustees, the assembly, nominations, and choices in the

APA that we liberalized very quickly. It was a very exciting time and the APA shifted significantly.

I studied the structure and constitution and bylaws of the APA—nearly no one had ever done that—and repeatedly wrote constitutional amendments; the CFCP proposed them by petition, and the APA membership passed them.

The board of trustees had been a rather closed and self-perpetuating circle of sixty-three-year-old white males, who wielded most APA power. I noticed that the APA was usually sluggish in taking any bold positions, partly because the board felt social issues were not adequately psychiatric and partly because of the APA Assembly, which tended to overrepresent the small and conservative states. (Wyoming, which had fourteen APA members, had the same APA Assembly representation as Manhattan, which had about 1,700 members.) When we helped the board become more socially active and liberal, in the early 1970s, there was an attempt at a sort of counterreformation, which tried to give the assembly ultimate power in the APA. That move, fortunately, failed.

While doing CFCP work nationally, I also began locally. I joined and soon became chair of the Social Issues Committee of the Northern New England (Massachusetts plus New Hampshire) Psychiatric Society. I was perceived as having reasonable values and lots of ideas, and the NNEPS was delighted that for a change somebody was trying to inject ideas into the APA. There had been, in most of Massachusetts' academic psychiatry, a fairly widespread disdain for (and ignorance about) the APA. However, a good many Bostonians and other New Englanders respected me, read some of what I wrote, listened, and decided that if I was doing it, it was probably okay. After some success with several other social issues, I asked Richard Pillard, who was in Boston and had recently become the only really openly gay psychiatrist that I knew, whether he and I could craft a several-point position paper, revising the psychiatric status of gayness, arguing that gayness was not an illness, and that gay people deserved full civil liberties. We thought, and think, that gayness does not meet decent criteria for a diagnosis or a mental illness. We produced a good draft, and got the NNEPS Social Issues Committee to discuss what a diagnosis is, and then to pass our draft. We then got the NNEPS Council to pass it, minus one or two small details, and send it on to the assembly. We eventually got the APA Assembly to discuss, think about the issues, identify with the cause a bit, and—somewhat to my surprise—to pass it. That grass-roots effort then joined the (simultaneous and more documented) parallel movement from the Committee on Nomenclature, the Council on Research, and the Reference Committee. To have the assembly educated and allied and even somewhat enthusiastic for this essentially scientific removal of homosexuality from the list of psychiatric diagnoses—that was politically timely, fortunate, and important for getting anything done. Even science is sometimes given opportunities by politics and timing. The wording that the APA finally used was our NNEPS wording, rather than the very similar wording from the Council on Research. I was one of several colleagues who worked on this. Several friends have generously suggested that my contributions included being right; writing (with Richard Pillard) a good draft; arguing and persuading well; sensing that the scientific and political climate was becoming right; helping analyze the steps needed and making the climate be right; helping to have several simultaneous psychiatric groups scientifically discuss, and then decide to change, the psychiatric status of homosexuality.

The vote by the APA Board of Trustees to remove homosexuality from the DSM in December 1973, was very gratifying. The board voted something like 13 to 0, with about three abstentions or absences, very heavily in favor of what we had helped to prepare. Some conservatives, largely psychoanalysts who did not like the board vote, tried to overturn it by a referendum of all APA members. That *failed,* though it muddied the waters somewhat: some reporters still say that the APA removed gayness from DSM-II by referendum, which is not true.

We were not aware at the time how important the APA 1973 decision would become.

JGLP: What did you do after that?

DR. HARTMANN: I went on seeing patients and teaching, and I became more and more active in general in the APA, and with many issues. I got myself elected to the APA Assembly—partly in order more forcefully to argue that the assembly, then less democratic and less efficient than the board, should have a large role but should not be the ultimate power in the APA. That was a major fight, and by a large APA membership vote, my side prevailed. The assembly then, to my pleasure and perhaps to its credit, despite my aggressively arguing that the assembly was not more democratic or efficient than the board, and despite my having been in the assembly only three years, promptly nominated me its speaker-elect. I was elected by a large majority, which was very gratifying; and I was unusually young at the time to be speaker, which was fun. I also worked for some child psychiatric organizations (AACAP [American Academy of Child and Adolescent Psychiatry], NECCAP [New England Council of Child and Adolescent Psychiatry]), and served on numerous APA committees and Councils. I helped get APA's GLB Caucus recognized, helped get the Committee on Gay, Lesbian, and Bisexual Issues established, helped get gay and lesbian representation in the assembly, helped that representation be heard and respected, and helped the APA to comment decently and thoughtfully on countless public policy and legal and social issues involving gayness and psychiatry. I was elected area trustee twice, then vice president, and then president of the APA.

I gave human rights a significant presence in the APA, and went on APA/human rights work trips to South Africa under apartheid, to Chile under Pinochet, and to the Soviet Union during their era of abuse of psychiatry and psychiatrists. I was, I think, known to be reasonably helpful and friendly, and loyal to the APA, and I tried to foster biopsychosocial integration and humane values.

One of my many issues remained, and remains, working out the ramifications of the 1973 decision. Psychiatry and psychoanalysis had been wrong about homosexuality, and had harmed gay people. I wanted psychiatry to be modest enough to change, to learn, and to do better. I became an internal presence for these ideas in APA leadership, and was also sometimes able to influence other organizations a bit, such as the American Psychological and the American Psychoanalytic [Associations].

JGLP: A lot has changed since then for gays.

DR. HARTMANN: Many things have changed over the last thirty, forty years. For instance, many people, including generally decent people, firmly thought that gay people should never be teachers, and that gay teachers should probably be fired. Many people—probably most—opposed gay adoption; that has changed, and much for the better. Gay foster-parenting was opposed as well. U.S. immigration rules treated gayness as a major contagious illness: it was flatly illegal to immigrate to this country if you were openly gay. (Not HIV positive. That was before HIV. Just gay.) Service in the military of course was an issue, with many discharges, and blackmail, and much hypocrisy. The area of so-called "reparative therapy," with its intrinsic harm to gay people and to psychiatry, demanded rethinking and change. Negative stereotypes abounded in all kinds of public places, including films and television: the nelly man, the bull dyke, the doomed gay relationship, the equation of gayness with pedophilia, the equation of gayness with major psychopathology and criminality, etc. All these areas, and more, APA gradually, over several decades, took as serious mental health issues and studied and wrote position papers and amicus briefs and letters about. APA helped change several U.S. government and state policies issues, including issues of ordinary civil rights: jobs, housing, health care decisions, access to health care, hospitalization visits, death arrangements, inheritance, and, recently very prominently, civil unions and gay marriage.

Much has changed, and the APA after 1973 frequently came forward to comment on gay issues from a now supportive point of view. That was far easier once the 1973 decision happened, and the APA was no longer trapped behind a pathologizing idea. It was also easier because an open and constructive gay presence was growing within the APA. I would also say—something that we did not anticipate in 1973—that the amount of good and thoughtful and many-sided literature on homosexuality—psychiatric and nonpsychiatric—published since 1973 has probably considerably exceeded the total amount of good and thoughtful literature on homosexuality written in the several thousand years before 1973.

JGLP: I heard that you officially came out at the end of your APA presidency. Is that true and could you talk about that?

DR. HARTMANN: To many people whom I do not know well, I think that is true. To family and friends, I had come out long before. To a great many other people, including many colleagues, I came out gradually over many years before that—gradually and often quietly, with some thought about pace and place, and in various degrees, because I wanted clearly to be known as a good, thoughtful, decent person, a good clinician and a sound teacher, and a politically and publicly sensible person. I tried to be, and to appear, a good and solid person, who is also gay.

Brian, my partner, and I have been together since early December 1973 (by coincidence, the month of the APA Board vote). We did a lot of ordinary things together, shared friends and gave parties together, and went to psychiatric and nonpsychiatric parties increasingly routinely together—but I did not invite Brian to come along to official APA functions until well into the 1980s. There was at that time, for instance, an annual APA officers' retreat, where about eight officers of the APA, their spouses, and about eight staff people got together for two or three days and talked about current psychiatric issues and who we were and what we wanted to do. As the new vice president, I decided that if I was going to be a good leader, and perhaps run for president, I had to be more explicitly open with all those people about myself and about living with Brian. So I brought Brian along, at APA expense, of course, as my partner, to an officers' retreat. I was anxious, but there was absolutely no trouble at all. The staff and others were respectful of (and perhaps even charmed by) Brian, and were pleased that I had the self-confidence or courage to do that.

In my increasingly public and visible APA life, there were occasional provocative questions, not all about gayness. While I was still in the assembly, for instance, after I had been noisily active on several social psychiatric issues, a curmudgeonly colleague asked a friend of mine, "Is Larry a Communist?" When I was on the board, another friend of mine, in California, was asked by a friend of his, "What's this outrageous idea that Dr. Hartmann may be gay and he's running for vice president?" My friend said, "I don't know the specifics about it, but what possible relevance could gayness have?"

When I did run for president two years later, a former APA Assembly colleague of mine—a dignified and conservative Southerner with whom I had disagreed politically on nearly every issue under the sun—wrote me a four-page letter of advice as to what I ought to do. At about page three, his letter said, "By the way, in the course of your running for president, I have heard that you may be gay. I have no idea what the truth of that is, but I certainly hope it won't impede your campaign for president, because I think you're just the kind of person who ought to be running the APA." That was gratifying.

While more and more people were aware of my gayness, I did not announce it as openly as some of my gay friends, especially younger gay friends, wanted me to, and I did not make it the central issue of my presidency. It remained *one* of my clear issues; I did speak about gay issues often, and I did appoint a disproportionate number of gay people to various positions.

APA presidents give two big speeches to the APA: one at the beginning, and a longer one at the end, of the presidential year. At the beginning of my year, I chose to be introduced, at the huge opening ceremony, by a good friend and mentor, Paul Fink, who was a past president. He asked if I wanted him to mention Brian. We talked about that for a while, and I said, "That's up to you. Only, if you do, I'd like to look at whatever words you say, so I can be comfortable with them." Paul decided, after a while, that he would not mention my living with Brian.

The next year I decided I would ask Mel Sabshin to introduce me; Mel was APA's medical director, and it was something of a favor, and not routine, for him to do that. He and I had worked together well and were friends, and I was glad also to be a friend of his wife's, before she died. He agreed to introduce me, as the outgoing president, and his remarks and my speech would, as is customary, be published in *AJP [American Journal of Psychiatry].* He also asked whether he should mention Brian. I said that I thought he should. We talked about how and what should he say about Brian and me, and he sent me some words, and I think I altered one or two of them. When I was then to give a speech to 2,500 psychiatrists at the opening ceremony, Mel Sabshin introduced me at some length in very flattering terms, and, with my full knowledge and cooperation, acknowledged my having shared my life for decades with Brian Pfeiffer, an architectural historian and social critic. Many people apparently heard that, and many others heard about it or later read it, and a good many let me know that they were glad. Several gay colleagues, at various stages of openness themselves, and several straight colleagues sent me "thank you" letters. I also was told by some people, as I'd half expected, "I wish you'd done that years before, and been more aggressive about it." (My partner, Brian, was among those who sometimes wished my pace of openness had been faster.)

Overall, one of the things that occurred to me was that different generations and half generations have been doing and will do openness about gayness in slightly different ways, and that is fine. (I expect that will include the next gay APA president.) I was gradual and rather quiet about it, but I was also consistently very much there and involved in fighting for social issues, including gay issues, for twenty or thirty years, openly and also behind the scenes.

JGLP: What are you working on now?

DR. HARTMANN: I see patients and continue my teaching at Harvard, and sit on a few boards of trustees. On the APA Board, I serve several functions, including, sometimes, a bit of institutional memory and social conscience. I teach mostly child and adolescent psychiatry. I also supervise residents. I have by now supervised a significant number of more or less openly gay residents, and that's remarkably different from what would have been possible a generation ago. I see patients in Cambridge, mostly adults but also children and adolescents. I see some couples. I have seen many gay patients (some of them colleagues) and many straight patients (some of them colleagues). I read, play tennis, swim, and climb not very challenging mountains.

I started something a few years ago with the Boston Psychoanalytic Institute, because I thought psychoanalysts were still remaining, more than psychiatrists in general, rather sluggish in their acceptance of and thoughtfulness about gayness. One of my tasks, because I am respectful of psychoanalysis, was to help the American Psychoanalytic [Association; APsaA] change, if I could; I raised gayness-and-psychoanalysis issues, and used my clout, such as it was, from 1988 through 1992, when I was APA VP, president-elect, and president, with APsaA leaders in our leaders' meetings. Because of my father, I had some slightly magical name recognition for APsaA leaders, which probably gave my issues some added interest for them. I nudged the APsaA somewhat, just at the time when Richard Isay was courageously acting to change the APsaA from within.

Anyway, in Boston in the 1990s, I had now and then urged several Boston analytic friends, for some years, to get the Boston Psychoanalytic [Institute] to accept openly gay candidates, and to rethink analysis and gayness, as was happening gradually here and there nationally. One friend, Gerry Adler, was president of the

Boston Psychoanalytic [Institute] at that time, and he and I started the Boston Psychoanalytic Group on Lesbian, Gay, Bisexual, and Transgender Issues. He and I continue to cochair that group. We have gotten some senior, middle-aged, and younger analysts and candidates involved, including two openly gay analytic candidates. We have had scientific meetings of various sizes and shapes—including, of course, presentations of gay-neutral or gay-positive analytic work—to help discuss and rethink gayness from a psychoanalytic point of view, and psychoanalysis from a gay point of view. Some of that occurs within BPSI [Boston Psychoanalytic Society and Institute]; some involves regular meetings of analysts with gay or gay-interested psychiatrists, psychologists, social workers, and others, in and around Boston. I think it has been useful.

JGLP: Any final thoughts?

DR. HARTMANN: I had very good fortune in growing up in a supportive and loving and friendly and highly educated family, and in having lots of good chances in life. I have also had the good fortune of growing up with an active social conscience. I wanted to work on a lot of scientific and artistic and social and political issues, and that came significantly to include gay issues, as gayness felt more and more authentic to me in my late teens and twenties and thirties. I am glad I have been able to do some useful work. I am very glad that I was able, even as a young psychiatrist, to contribute in some ways that used who I am reasonably well from several points of view—to help contribute to the 1973 change; and then to get myself into a position where I could help to organize psychiatry to be supportive and creative in helping develop further changes over the next thirty-plus years. That is something I am pleased about.

I feel good about many things in my career and life, but I am particularly pleased that I have been able to be an active part of a time when the status of gayness has changed dramatically and usefully for the better. As I said in my introduction to the *Textbook of Homosexuality*,[4] the historic cultural conceptual change from seeing gayness as a *sin* to seeing it as a *crime* to seeing it as an *illness* to seeing it as a *difference* is a huge change. That change is still very difficult for many people to understand and integrate and accept. I think it is important to go on working on that. In general, especially in areas of prejudice, irrational traditions, and strong feelings, I think that as psychiatrists and citizens we have to work in whatever ways we can at helping people consolidate the idea that different does not mean better or worse. It often means interesting.

Psychiatrists should respect and enjoy diversity, and be careful not to impose societal disapprovals as if they were diagnostic labels. We have learned something about that.

There are many people to whom I am grateful, certainly including my partner, Brian, my family and friends, my patients, my teachers, my students; colleagues I have worked with in the APA, at Harvard, and elsewhere; colleagues who helped with the 1973 decision, including Judd Marmor and Evelyn Hooker, both of whom died recently; and not least, you and other colleagues who are continuing to do energetic and useful work for gayness and for psychiatry.[5]

NOTES

1. Heinz Hartman, MD, is also known as the father of American ego psychology. See Hartmann, H. (1958), *Ego Psychology and the Problem of Adaptation*, trans. D. Rapaport. New York: International Universities Press.

2. Formerly Boston Psychopathic Hospital.

3. See Bayer, R. (1981), *Homosexuality and American Psychiatry: The Politics of Diagnosis*. New York: Basic Books; and David Scasta's article on John E. Fryer, MD, and the Dr. H. Anonymous episode, Chapter 1 in this book.

4. Cabaj, R.P. & Stein, T.S., eds. (1996), *Textbook of Homosexuality and Mental Health*. Washington, DC: American Psychiatric Press.

5. This interview was prepared in 2003 and 2004.

SELECTED BIBLIOGRAPHY

Doerr, O., Hartmann, L., Lira, E. & Weinstein, E. (1972), Torture: Phenomenology and psychiatric sequelae. *Psychiatry,* 55(5):177-184.

Hartmann, L. (1973), Some uses of dirty words by children. *J. Amer. Acad. Child & Adolesc. Psychiat.,* 12(1):108-122.

Hartmann, L. & Hanson, G. (1986), Child psychotherapy. In: *Current Psychiatric Therapies,* ed. J. Masserman. New York: Grune and Stratton, pp. 29-43.

Nightingale, E., Hartmann, L., Hannibal, K., Geiger, J., Lawrence, R. & Spurlock, J. (1990), Apartheid medicine. *JAMA,* 264(16):2097-2102.

Hartmann, L. (1991), Humane values and bio-psychosocial integration. *Amer. J. Psychiat.,* 148(3):1130-1134.

Hartmann, L. (1992a), Some social psychiatric problems in Chile, South Africa and the Soviet Union. In: *Psychiatry and World Accords,* ed. J. Masserman. New York, Gardner, pp. 5-15.

Hartmann, L. (1992b), Reflections on humane values and bio-psychosocial integration. *Amer. J. Psychiat.,* 149(9):1135-1144.

Hartmann, L. (1994), Heinz Hartmann: A memorial tribute and filial memoir. *Psychoanal. Study of the Child,* 49:3-12.

Hanson, G. & Hartmann, L. (1996), Latency development in prehomosexual boys. In: *Textbook of Homosexuality and Mental Health,* ed. R.P. Cabaj & T.S. Stein. Washington, DC: American Psychiatric Press, pp. 253-266.

Hartmann, L. (1996), Foreword. In: *Textbook of Homosexuality and Mental Health,* ed. R.P. Cabaj & T.S. Stein. Washington, DC: American Psychiatric Press, pp. xxv-xxxi.

Hartmann, L. (1998a), Children are left out. *Amer. J. Forensic Psychiat.,* 19(3): 33-44.

Hartmann, L. (1998b), Eros in a gay dyad: A discussion. *Gender & Psychoanalysis,* 3(3)361-371.

Hartmann, L. (1998c), Physician-assisted suicide. *Psychiatric Services,* 49(11):1468-1474.

Hartmann, L. (2001), Confidentiality. In: *Primer of the APA,* ed. D. Langsley. Washington, DC: American Psychiatric Press, pp. 39-45.

Hartmann, L. (2003), Too flawed; Don't publish: A commentary on Spitzer and changing sexual orientation. *Archives Sexual Behavior,* 32:436-438.

Chapter 4

An Interview with Robert Jean Campbell III, MD

Richard O. Hire

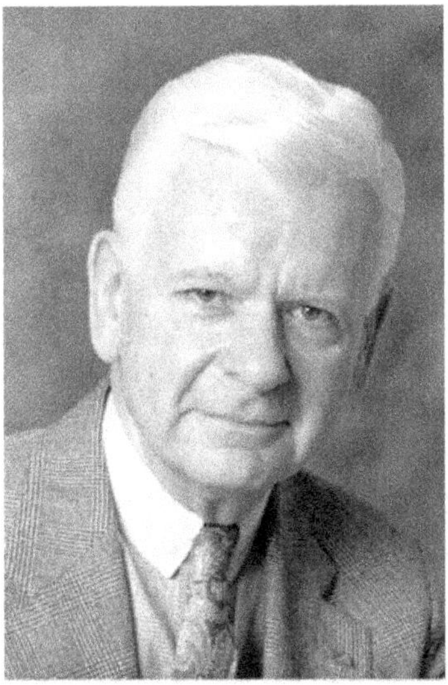

I met with Dr. Robert J. Campbell on a sunny afternoon in early May 2000. We spoke for several hours in the living room of his elegant apartment on the Upper East Side of Manhattan where he resides with Cesare Santeramo, his partner of thirty-four years.

In a career spanning five decades, Dr. Campbell has made important contributions to psychiatry encompassing many areas. These include medical education and research, organizational and administrative psychiatry, and community psychiatry. He has served in numerous important legislative and executive positions at all levels of organized psychiatry and has been an early and energetic advocate for the profession and our patients in the political and public arenas. He is currently Clinical Professor of Psychiatry at Cornell University Medical College, and has been the Medical Director of Gracie Square Hospital in New York City since 1977. His publications include over

This chapter appeared originally under the same title in *Journal of Gay & Lesbian Psychotherapy* 6(3):81-96. Copyright 2002 The Haworth Press, Inc.

doi:10.1300/6049_05

150 books, chapters, articles, and reviews (an abbreviated bibliography of his publications is included at the end of this interview). He is probably most widely known for *Campbell's Psychiatric Dictionary,* and was working on the eighth edition when we met. He was for many years the Editor-in-Chief of the American Psychiatric Association's *Psychiatric News,* as well as Editor-in-Chief of the New York State Psychiatric Association's newsletter, *The Bulletin.* Dr. Campbell also serves on the boards of many philanthropic organizations and is the recipient of many national and international awards recognizing his contributions to psychiatry, the arts, and international human rights. At the time of our interview I was glad to see he was still going strong.

JGLP: The *Journal of Gay & Lesbian Psychotherapy* is publishing a series of biographical interviews which includes pioneers in psychiatry who have made important contributions to gay and lesbian patients and their therapists. I know you have played many important roles in the American Psychiatric Association (APA) over the years. In Bayer's 1981 book[1] about the efforts to remove the diagnosis of homosexuality from the *Diagnostic and Statistical Manual,* you are mentioned as being involved in that effort. The book describes what sounds like a tumultuous time in the APA.

DR. CAMPBELL: Yes, a lot of things were going on at that time. This was the period when a feminist interrupted a speaker at the annual meeting and got on the stage to speak herself, and he said, "You bitch, get off my program!" Things were really bad. We anticipated lots of physical assaults. All sorts of antipsychiatry movements came during that time. They would come to the annual meeting and fly banners saying, "PSYCHIATRY KILLS." Then one of our own members began to bring this banner against ECT [electroconvulsive therapy] and tried to get that outlawed. That was a big political issue for a long time. Then the issue about homosexuality came up. It divided the association and they finally had to have a referendum. Imagine calling a referendum on what is a scientific issue! Fortunately, there were a few scientists who prevailed. The board of trustees was, to me, surprisingly open about this. I expected much more opposition.

JGLP: Were you on the board at that time?

DR. CAMPBELL: No. This was back in 1973. I think. I was on the board from 1983 to 1990.

JGLP: In his book, Bayer mentions that you had contact with the group of gay activists, offering to bring the diagnostic question to the APA in order to try and get some communication going.

DR. CAMPBELL: Yes. I was in Washington for a meeting of the assembly. At that point, the activist group of five members—led by Frank Kameny who was a social worker—heard the APA was meeting in Washington. They didn't understand that this was the meeting of the assembly, and not the APA Board. I was a member of the APA Committee on Nomenclature and Statistics, and the only member of the committee to be a member of the assembly. I was there on assembly work and they discovered that I was also a member of the committee.

They called me out of nowhere to say, "We think that psychiatry is mistreating homosexuals terribly and we want you to do something about it." I said, "Me! What can I do?" I don't think they asked me on the basis of knowing I was gay. I think they asked on the basis that this would have to be part of the official nomenclature if it were to change, and I just happened to be the one who was there.

Well, it was a funny meeting. Frank Kameny, I thought, was rather strange and quite difficult. Fortunately the others were calmer. Charles Silverstein was especially good and the most sensible person in the group. He was a psychologist and he knew the technical language. They made a presentation that went on for maybe two hours and it was very convincing. They had a lot of data that I had never seen. I don't know where they got it, but I was really overwhelmed by the data. I said in all sincerity that I would do everything that I possibly could to arrange for this issue to come up for official review.

Our committee on Nomenclature met a month later in New York. By then, I had served four years as a member of my eight-year term. The chairman was a nice elder statesman from one of the state hospitals on Long Island. Another member was Bill Langford, Chief of Pediatric Psychiatry at Columbia. Another man was from Washington. The newest member was Robert Spitzer. So I brought up the issue of homosexuality and said if we are going to call this a disease, maybe we should be sure we knew all of the recent scientific findings about the particular issue. Well, it met with some resistance. The heaviest resistance was from Spitzer. Langford, being a child psychiatrist, was more accustomed to these things and said he thought it would be interesting to review. And then, oddly enough, the next youngest member (Spitzer was the youngest), who I thought might be quite reactionary, said, "Yes, why don't we have a look at all of that and maybe we could even talk to them." I said, "I think they would really appreciate that."

So we had a meeting and the activist group came. They presented pretty much the same material they had presented to me. Everyone except Spitzer expressed interest. We discussed it among ourselves and I tried to be as objective as possible because I thought it would be politically unwise to take a very pro-homosexual position if it later became common knowledge that I was homosexual. I didn't want them to think that I was making my point because it referred to me. I tried to walk a careful line between self-interest and objectivity. So I suggested that we have a subgroup of the committee to research the literature and come back to report on the scientific findings about the subject. They agreed that was a good idea.

Needless to say I wanted Dr. Spitzer on the committee. He was the youngest member and I thought should do the work, and I also thought if he worked with someone who had a calming effect, maybe he wouldn't be so difficult. Well, it worked. I put him on with the other younger member who had been fairly open to the idea of looking at the question. I thought they were enough the same age, they'll talk the same language. They were our committee of two.

JGLP: Do you recall the other member's name?

DR. CAMPBELL: No. His name may have been Wilson but I'm not sure. They did the research and came back and said, "You know, those guys are much more solid in what they have been saying from a scientific viewpoint than what our official position has been. We think we should bring this to the board." So we brought it to the Board of Trustees of the APA. I think, but can't remember for sure, that the board also heard the presentation from the gay group. After a little nudging of some board members, it was brought to a vote, and it was decided to take homosexuality out of the DSM as a disorder. Then there were many objections from "our friends" in New York City.

JGLP: Are you referring to the psychoanalysts?

DR. CAMPBELL: I thought the only reason they were worried was that they wouldn't have any patients if this went through. People would no longer go to them for something that was no longer a disease. I must say, I hadn't anticipated that would happen. So the idea of a referendum was proposed by them.

JGLP: How did that come about?

DR. CAMPBELL: It was through the efforts of Bieber and Socarides and their group. I had known Bieber and he had a kind of neutral respect for me—not much but some. Socarides and I would get in the same room and sparks would fly! He had an ability to misinterpret things. I was amazed this ended up in a referendum. Some of the things the association went through to make this palatable were rather funny. The analysts said there are some homosexuals who need some help when they go through an identity crisis and that sort of thing. So they invented a diagnosis called "sexual orientation disturbance" which got published.[2] This made them happy until somebody pointed out that "sexual orientation disorder of male youths" spelled "sodomy." So they decided this diagnosis was not such a good out. I was also on the glossary committee and we worked out a definition that did away with sexual orientation disturbance disorder. Anyone can have identity disturbance disorder for any number of reasons, so over the years it was toned down.[3] So anyway, we got homosexuality out of the DSM. I don't think there has been any back-tracking on this decision in the APA, although there hasn't been as much forward movement as I would have hoped. I think the majority of medical schools are no longer biased against homosexuality as far as admissions policy.

JGLP: Do you feel your homosexuality has affected your career?

DR. CAMPBELL: Early in my career, I was as brainwashed as everybody else at the time in thinking that one had to become an analyst, at least in New York. I made all of the preparations and went through, I think, six interviews. By the way, in two of these interviews, the analysts who were judging my appropriateness for their profession fell asleep while I was talking to them! I mean they didn't even have me on the couch. We were face-to-face! This did not please me at all. I'm not one to let my thoughts or feelings lie secret. I'm told I should never play poker because what I'm thinking is obvious on my face when all my cards are down. I must have transmitted my feelings somehow because all six of them found me "not appropriate for analytic training." Well, I knew from the tenor of the questions what it was that put at least some of them off. One of them asked how I spent my free time on the weekend. I said, "Well, my wife and I go up to our place in the country." And he said, "Your wife! Oh, I didn't realize you were married." And I said, "Yes. Would you like to know how many children I have? I have two." Anyway, I knew perfectly well what it was that put them off, that they considered homosexuals sick, deviant, and unworthy of this high calling.

I don't think I was affected in other ways so much, although I'm told it affected my run for the presidency of the APA. I'm told that my rival made no bones about the fact that I was gay.

JGLP: Were you "out" about your sexuality during that time?

DR. CAMPBELL: Oh, yes. I talked about it in public addresses during the campaign.

JGLP: Who was your opponent?

DR. CAMPBELL: I don't recall his name. He was from California. I had two rivals at different times. There are only two people who ever ran twice for the APA presidency and lost, Robert Michels and myself. The second time I lost to George Tarjan by I think twenty-three votes, but he was a recognized man in the field and had worked very hard for the APA. He had run once before and lost. I didn't mind losing that race so much.

JGLP: What are some of your memories running for the president of the APA?

DR. CAMPBELL: I must admit I was a little uncomfortable about the gay issue. I knew perfectly well that it was a problem for some. Here in New York, I remember going to Middletown or someplace upstate, to talk about legislative issues, and the question of the referendum on homosexuality in the DSM came up. And it was clear that that district branch would have voted with the old guard. I knew it would be a problem in the election. I also knew that I'm not a good politician in the sense of all of a sudden making myself believable to people that I never had anything to do with. So all the other minority groups who generally get behind the minority candidate were not necessarily in my corner. I couldn't go to the Indians and say, "I'm basically Indian." I'd never talked with them before. I hadn't been particularly pro-feminist. I thought what the feminists were doing to the language was ridiculous, that you had to say "he/she" all the time. I thought it was so cumbersome. There were many women who supported me, Elisa Benedek among others, but I can't say I got the women's vote. Also, I've always been rather open about my feelings about children. In medical school, every time I picked up a baby it would shit or pee on me. I couldn't stand it!

JGLP: So you weren't good at kissing babies?

DR. CAMPBELL: I wasn't good at kissing babies, so I didn't get the child and adolescent group vote. I didn't pick up the number of votes that one minority might expect to pick up from the other minorities.

JGLP: I know you have been active in the APA for many years. What are some of the positions you've held and some of the other things that you've accomplished?

DR. CAMPBELL: Well, I've been vice president of the APA. I was on the board of trustees for eight years and i was the speaker of the assembly. I was one of five members who formed the Joint Commission on Government Relations, and as soon as it became organized, I became the first chairman. Under my leadership, we formed the Corporation for the Advancement of Psychiatry, and spun off from that the Political Action Committee. I'm still the president of the corporation and the chairman of the Political Action Committee.

I've done a lot of writing for the APA. I've been involved in all the editions of the *American Psychiatric Glossary* since the second edition. I wrote a monograph for the APA on *Psychiatry and Primary Care Physicians*. I've been the editor-in-chief of *Psychiatric News* from 1983 until 1998. I was editor-in-chief of *The Bulletin,* which is the newsletter of the New York State Psychiatric Association, from 1982 to 1997, and I was associate editor from 1964-1982. I have also been involved in public affairs and public relations for the association, starting with the New York County District Branch, then as public information officer for the Area II [New York State] Council, and I was one of the earliest public information officers for the APA itself. I had been doing public affairs under a different name for seven years before the APA finally formed the Joint Commission on Public Affairs. I'd been involved because I felt that psychiatry was very misunderstood by the public and certainly by legislators, who I saw were beginning—via legislation—to move into the actual practice of medicine. So I thought the thing to do was to educate the legislators. That's why I stayed so involved in legislative affairs, not because, as I said, I'm a politician, because I'm not. I thought of it as an educational effort. And I tried to keep in touch with the media as regularly as I could to get us positive exposure. Clearly there is still much work to be done in this area.

JGLP: I recall that you were an early advocate of the medical underpinnings of psychiatry.

DR. CAMPBELL: Before I became medical director at Gracie Square, I worked at St. Vincent's Hospital. Harvey Tompkins was our chair then and he was very big in the APA. Those were the days in the APA when there was one nominating slate and your buddies put you in and you knew five years in advance when you would be president. Harvey was so proud of the fact that when he was elected so many people voted, not that they voted for him—because there was no choice—but that so many voted. This was taken as a sign of great achievement! I was fairly close with Harvey. He was not very interested in writing, and I wrote a lot of his material for him. I'm not sure some of the time that he understood what I was writing because it wasn't really consistent with his philosophy!

Anyway, one day he came back from a meeting in Washington and said, "Come out to lunch. I have something to tell you about that you'll really be happy about." So we went out to lunch, and he told me how pleased I would be to know that we had managed to split psychiatry off from neurology and we were now going to have the *Archives of Psychiatry* as a separate publication from the *Archives of Neurology*. I said, "Harvey, I would never have suggested that! We're trying to go in the opposite direction!" He said, "You mean you don't think that's a good move?" I said, "It's terrible! Why couldn't you at least leave sleeping dogs lie!" Well, my whole approach is that we are a great part of neurology and should never have split off. And what we are now discovering, of course, is that we should have learned more neurology and kept it in our minds all these years because we are coming back to it. So, anyway, my philosophy was a little different from what was prevalent in New York City at the time.

JGLP: I know you've edited or written over 150 books, articles, and reviews. *Campbell's Psychiatric Dictionary* is the best known to many. How did you get started with the dictionary?

DR. CAMPBELL: It's still selling! When I was a student at Columbia, Leland Hinsie was second-in-command in the department. He and a librarian, Jacob Shatzky, had thought up the idea and wrote the original dictionary in 1940. It was heavily oriented to the old descriptions of clinical patients, and the new psychoanalytic theories of what those descriptions meant. It was a funny combination. Shatzky knew nothing about psychiatry. His claim to fame was that he was an avid follower of book sales, and he happened to notice that a particular private library was for sale. He recognized from his knowledge of libraries in general that this must be Freud's library. So with Columbia's funds, he brought Freud's collection into Columbia's library and became famous for that. What he did in the dictionary were the derivations. For example, under "Medea complex," he wrote two paragraphs on who Medea was, and under "Oedipus complex," he had four paragraphs, all of which were filler pages really. He and Hinsie didn't have enough definitions to work with. They then brought out a second edition, which actually wasn't a full book. It was meant to be appended to the first edition. It was during the war and paper was expensive; labor was not available. So instead of taking this new group of definitions and putting it in the first edition, they published it as an addendum but called it Volume II.

It so happened that I was a medical student at Columbia at that time, and I was in Dr. Hinsie's class. He said he was doing this dictionary and asked if anyone would be interested. I won't go into why I was interested, but I had become a rabid reader of Samuel Johnson, the eighteenth-century lexicographer and author of *Dictionary of the English Language.* I said I was interested. I was a resident before it was time to come up with any definitions. He had about twelve original collaborators from medical school and out of those, only I and one other remained as collaborators. Hinsie was not a stylist and he recognized it was kind of an uneven addition, but the second edition came out, published by Oxford University Press in 1953.

I became the editor in 1956. Dr. Hinsie was a man with many interests. He had a great big office, where he kept a stock market ticker which he watched avidly. He and a pathologist friend were both interested in the market. In 1956 they hit the jackpot. I don't know which stock it was, but he announced he was now rich enough to retire, so he did. He called Oxford and said he would no longer be editor for the dictionary, but said he had a new editor, Robert Campbell. And he told them he wouldn't relinquish the editorship until they told him that I would be editor.

It was 1956 and the third edition was due in 1957. He didn't give me anything written after the second edition so I had a year to get this done. I gave up my vacation. I took a house in Amagansett and spent the entire three months doing nothing but writing definitions. But I got it done. I had to be careful because many of the collaborators were still alive and you have no idea about the narcissistic investment that a writer gives to every word that appears on the page. So I had to be very careful in trimming and editing.

I'm presently working on the eighth edition. The seventh edition came out in 1995. We get out a new edition about every six or seven years. Oxford would like it to come out more frequently because it is their best seller in the science market. I do enjoy doing the dictionary and it makes me stay current with areas of study I might not otherwise read about. I've written glossaries for other texts and I've been co-editor of the *American Psychiatric Glossary* for the APA. I'm a member of the Dictionary Society of North America and we have abstruse meetings from time to time.

JGLP: In addition to organized, administrative, and academic psychiatry, I know you have also been involved in community psychiatry and especially the Alcoholism Council of New York.

DR. CAMPBELL: Yes, for a long time. It was kind of a fluke how I got involved. They were looking for someone in medicine familiar with drugs and medications. Some on the council were enlightened enough to see that the split that AA [Alcoholics Anonymous] originally made between alcohol and the use of medication was not very appropriate because so many people with alcoholism had comorbid illnesses which needed treatment and treatment often included medication. St. Vincent's Hospital was very close by, so they picked me for geographical reasons, I think.

There was a very dynamic CEO of the Alcoholism Council, Bill Plunket. He was very bright and knowledgeable. He didn't have the rigid attitude that if you are an alcoholic you can never have another drink. He wasn't that kind of AA person. I liked him and I liked working with him. So, we got to talking and I saw the problems they were having were similar to the problems that psychiatry was having and had been having. The public doesn't really know what alcoholism is about. This was before the days it was recognized as a disease. The definition of an alcoholic was that you drank more than your doctor did; that was the level of diagnostic sophistication.

We decided one problem was that nothing was really taught about alcoholism in medical school. Over a period of years, we decided one major focus should be to try to get the medical schools in New York to start talking about alcoholism and training clinicians to treat it. If you wanted an illness that had multiple modes of presentation, you couldn't pick a better one.

I went around trying to sell this idea to the medical schools. Many worried they would end up with a bunch of drunks in their emergency rooms and didn't want any part of it. I kept urging them to give it a try and at Columbia they did, probably to humor me. They had a series of grand rounds on Saturdays and they let me appear with some other people and we had an annual program. We had many interesting speakers: a famous author and various researchers on alcoholism and liver specialists (back then everyone equated liver disease with cirrhosis from alcohol). It became a well-known program. I remember a celebrity or two who were interested in alcoholism who attended. The program went on for several years. Then the idea of teaching about alcoholism gradually spread. Cornell started a program, then New York University, and we really started to get somewhere.

JGLP: It seems to me that you've confronted bias on a number of fronts during your career.

DR. CAMPBELL: You are right. I have always been upset when people reach a conclusion about something about which they know none of the facts that should have preceded their conclusion. I started with the Council on Alcoholism around 1968 and became chairman of the training program. We decided that if we couldn't get the medical schools to teach about alcoholism (which they didn't at first), then we could develop a training program to take into a social agency and train them and then have them train other agencies.

So we formed a team and I was the physician and director. After that, I was asked to join the board in the 1970s and was elected chairman around 1987. I was the first physician to serve as chairman.

JGLP: Can you tell me something about your early life and how you decided to become a psychiatrist?

DR. CAMPBELL: I was born in Wisconsin and lived there until I was thirteen. I left in 1939. I was bored with school, skipped the eighth grade, and finished high school in three years. I was bored there, too, except I liked it better because I was in boarding school and away from my parents. By the second day there, I remember thinking that these were the first two happy days I'd ever had in my life. It was very dramatic at the time and I only returned home for brief vacations after that. I sometimes have little sympathy for people who talk about the grief and anxiety children have upon separation from their parents. I found it relieved my anxiety enormously. My father was very strict. I entered the University of Wisconsin and because of the pressures of wartime was able to finish my undergraduate degree in three years. So I was eighteen years old when I began medical school and twenty-two when I graduated. Fortunately, I was tall for my age so no one knew how much younger I was and it didn't bother me.

I was studying under the psychologist Harry Harlow at the University of Wisconsin and thought that I would become a psychologist. At the time, I hadn't even considered clinical psychology. I got involved in a series of studies that had to do with frontal lobotomies in the rhesus monkey. This was in 1943. Although various people are taking credit for observing it nowadays, he and I observed that, following frontal lobotomies, the monkeys had a restless pacing circular activity, a stereotypic activity, which we described and published. Some of the neurologists that worked with us considered this to be a significant observation, as it seemed to pinpoint where stereotypy could be traced.

I was only seventeen and very naive at the time. The research got good reviews from psychologists but little notice from people dealing with patients. So I thought if they wouldn't pay any attention to me doing this research, I'll go to medical school. So that was how I decided on medical school. I went to Columbia. I had applied to several schools and was turned down by Harvard and Johns Hopkins—and I think Yale. But Columbia accepted me.

JGLP: Were you working on a PhD in psychology?

DR. CAMPBELL: I was working on my master's. What happened was that the draft [for the armed services] came in and I didn't want to wait to get my PhD before I went on to my medical studies, so I just dropped everything in psychology and went off the following June to Columbia.

JGLP: Did you know you wanted to be a psychiatrist when you started medical school?

DR. CAMPBELL: Well, I knew I didn't want to be a surgeon! I can remember very well the day we started there. We started early in June. In the physiology course, they had just learned this new technique from the Russians: to drain a dog's blood out so that it was dead and then put it back in. I was sitting in the middle of the room watching this. The blood flowed copiously in the beginning, but toward the end it went drip, drip, drip. And with each drip I began to feel more and more uncomfortable until I passed out. I woke up in the hallway with three women from my medical class ministering to me! I was like that with blood all the way through medical school. By the time I got to the surgery rotation, my first assignment was in obstetrics and gynecology. My first surgical experience was with a woman who had to have a Caesarian section. As the lowest one on the totem pole, I was given the retractors and hemostats. They hadn't warned me about the amount of bleeding in this procedure. When the blood spurted all over, I of course fell to the ground, taking all the instruments with me! As you can understand, the surgeon could have killed me. So I realized that surgery was not going to be my specialty.

I wasn't sure I would go into psychiatry. I was debating between psychiatry, neurology, and internal medicine from the point of view of a diagnostician, of knowing where to send people rather than knowing how to take care of them. But what I think tipped me toward psychiatry was that nobody seemed to know anything. It was clear to me as a student that all of these people had wonderful theories, but there was not one shred of evidence. I mean it was all anecdotal. I thought this was not a very scientific area, and maybe it needs a little shaking up. I don't mind nonclosure. There are lots of things one doesn't know. So that's what intrigued me about psychiatry. And of course in the back of my mind was also the thought that maybe I would get back to what had got me onto all this in the first place, my frontal lobotomy experiments.

JGLP: Looking back on your career and life up to this point, what do you think has been your greatest contribution?

DR. CAMPBELL: I think probably the dictionary. As the second, I would put teaching. I've always enjoyed teaching and have always had an enormously positive response from students, and continue to hear from many former students even today.

JGLP: It's interesting you mention your teaching. I remember the first time I heard your name mentioned, when I first moved to New York many years ago, was from a social worker who had been your student at St. Vincent's Hospital and who told me what an exceptional and memorable teacher you were for her. Thank you for spending this time with me and sharing so much history.

NOTES

1. Bayer, R. (1981), *Homosexuality and American Psychiatry: The Politics of Diagnosis.* New York: Basic Books.

2. Editor's Note: The diagnosis of "homosexuality" was replaced by "sexual orientation disturbance" in the DSM-II.

3. Editor's Note: In 1980, "sexual orientation disturbance" was changed to "ego-dystonic homosexuality" in the DSM-III. The latter diagnosis was eventually removed from the DSM-III-R(evised) in 1987. For a report on that decision, see Krajeski, J. (1996), Homosexuality and the mental health professions. In: *Textbook of Homosexuality and Mental Health,* ed. R. P. Cabaj & T. S. Stein. Washington, DC: American Psychiatric Press, pp. 17-31.

SELECTED BIBLIOGRAPHY

Books and Book Chapters

Campbell, R. J., collaborator (1953), *Hinsie and Shatsky's Psychiatric Dictionary,* Second Edition. New York: Oxford University Press.

Campbell, R. J. (1960), *Hinsie and Campbell's Psychiatric Dictionary,* Third Edition. New York: Oxford University Press.

Campbell, R. J. (1962), The etiology and background of chronic alcoholism. In: *Problems in Addiction,* ed. W. Bier. New York: Fordham University Press, pp. 59-70.

Campbell, R. J. (1962), Psychiatric factors in addiction. In: *Problems in Addiction,* ed. W. Bier. New York: Fordham University Press, pp. 165-170.

Campbell, R. J. (1963), Masturbation and homosexuality. In: *The Adolescent: His Search for Understanding,* ed. W. Bier. New York: Fordham University Press, pp. 52-61.

Campbell, R. J. (1964), Adolescent sexual development. In: *Personality and Sexual Problems in Pastoral Psychology,* ed. W. Bier. New York: Fordham University Press, pp. 137-151.

Campbell, R. J. (1967), Facilitation of short-term clinic therapy. In: *Current Psychiatric Therapies,* Volume VII, ed. J. H. Masserman. New York: Grune and Stratton, pp. 186-196.

Campbell, R. J. (1968), Why women do not marry. In: *Woman in Modern Life,* ed. W. Bier. New York: Fordham University Press, pp. 183-193.

Campbell, R. J. (1969), Increasing validity of biochemical studies in mental disorders. In: *The Future of the Brain Sciences,* ed. S. Bogock. New York: Plenum Press, pp. 571-573.

Campbell, R. J. (1970), *Hinsie and Campbell's Psychiatric Dictionary,* Fourth Edition. New York: Oxford University Press.

Campbell, R. J. (1970), Lithium: A review. In: *Out-Patient Psychiatry in the 1970's,* ed. A. Tulipan & D. Heyder. New York: Brunner/Mazel, pp. 89-97.

Campbell, R. J. (1970), *Psychiatric Education and the Primary Physician.* Washington, DC: American Psychiatric Association.

Campbell, R. J. (1972), Alienation and homosexuality. In: *Alienation: Plight of Modern Man?,* ed. W. Bier. New York: Fordham University Press, pp. 219-229.

Campbell, R. J. (1974), Psychopathology of aging. In: *Aging: Its Challenge to the Individual and to Society,* ed. W. Bier. New York: Fordham University Press, pp. 96-116.

Frazier, S. H., Campbell, R. J., Marshall, M. & Werner, A., ed. (1975), *A Psychiatric Glossary,* Fourth Edition. Washington, DC: American Psychiatric Association.

Werner, A., Campbell, R. J., Frazier, S. H. & Stone, E., eds. (1980), *A Psychiatric Glossary,* Fifth Edition. Washington, DC: American Psychiatric Association.

Campbell, R. J. (1981), *Campbell's Psychiatric Dictionary,* Fifth Edition. New York: Oxford University Press.

Campbell, R. J. (1981), The nosology of psychiatry. In: *American Handbook of Psychiatry,* Volume VII, ed. S. Arieti & H. K. H. Brodie. New York: Basic Books, pp. 649-671.

Campbell, R. J. (1985), Lessons for the future drawn from United States legislation and experience. In: *Psychiatry, Human Rights and the Law,* ed. M. Roth & R. Bluglass. Cambridge: Cambridge University Press, pp. 43-57.

Campbell, R. J. (1985), Miscellaneous organic therapies. In: *Comprehensive Textbook of Psychiatry,* Fourth Edition, ed. H. I. Kaplan and B. J. Sadock. Baltimore, MD: Williams and Wilkins, pp. 1569-1575.

Campbell, R. J., ed. for Psychiatry (1986), *International Dictionary of Medicine and Biology.* New York: John Wiley & Sons.

Campbell, R. J. (1989), *Campbell's Psychiatric Dictionary,* Sixth Edition. New York: Oxford University Press.

Campbell, R. J., ed. for Psychiatry (1989), *Churchill's Medical Dictionary.* New York: Churchill Livingstone.

Campbell, R. J. & Edgerton, J. E., eds. (1994), *American Psychiatric Glossary.* Washington, DC: American Psychiatric Press, Inc.

Babor, T., Campbell, R. J., Room, R. & Saunders, J., compilers (1994), *Lexicon of Alcohol and Drug Terms.* Geneva: World Health Organization.

Campbell, R. J., Jablensky, A. & Shepherd, M., eds. (1994), *Lexicon of Psychiatric and Mental Health Terms,* Second Edition. Geneva: World Health Organization.

Campbell, R. J. (1996), *Psychiatric Dictionary,* Seventh Edition. New York: Oxford University Press.

Campbell, R. J. (2000), Managed care. In: *Comprehensive Textbook of Psychiatry,* Seventh Edition, ed. B. J. Sadock & V. S. Sadock. Baltimore, MD: Williams and Wilkins, pp. 3199-3209.

Articles

Campbell, R. J. & Harlow, H. F. (1945), Problem solution by monkeys following bilateral removal of the prefrontal area V. spatial delayed reactions. *J. Experimental Psychology,* 35:110-126.

Campbell, R. J. (1958), The schizophrenias—Current views. *Psychiatric Quarterly,* 32:318-334.

Zane, M. D. & Campbell, R. J. (1962), Course on psychiatry for physicians. *New York State Journal of Medicine,* 62:3430-3434.

Tompkins, H. J. & Campbell, R. J. (1966), Brief psychotherapy. *Proceedings, IV World Congress of Psychiatry.* Madrid, Spain, pp. 407-415.

Campbell, R. J. (1966), Clinical application of research in psychotherapy. *Mental Hygiene,* 50:580-583.

Campbell, R. J., Scolaro, M. & Bogoch, S. (1967), Cerebrospinal fluid glycoproteins in schizophrenia. *Amer. J. Psychiat.,* 123:952-962.

Campbell, R. J. (1978), Report of the speaker-elect. *Amer. J. Psychiat.,* 135:1292-1293.

Campbell, R. J. (1979), Report of the speaker. *Amer. J. Psychiat.,* 136:1380-1382.

Campbell, R. J. (1981), The language of psychiatry. *Hospital & Community Psychiatry,* 32:849-852.

Campbell, R. J. (1983), The mentally ill: Struggles of psychiatric patients for access to care. *Bulletin, New York Academy of Medicine,* 59:50-58.

Campbell, R. J. (1984), Flashbacks: Scenes from psychiatry's revolutions. *Bulletin, New York Academy of Medicine,* 60:479-493.

Campbell, R. J. (1985), The psychiatrist as physician. *Psychosomatics,* 26:48-54.
Campbell, R. J. (1986), An overdose of peer review? *Hospital and Community Psychiatry,* 37:111.
Campbell, R. J. (1986), The triangle of health care. *Psychiatric Quarterly,* 58:15-23.

Chapter 5

An Interview with Judd Marmor, MD

Vernon A. Rosario

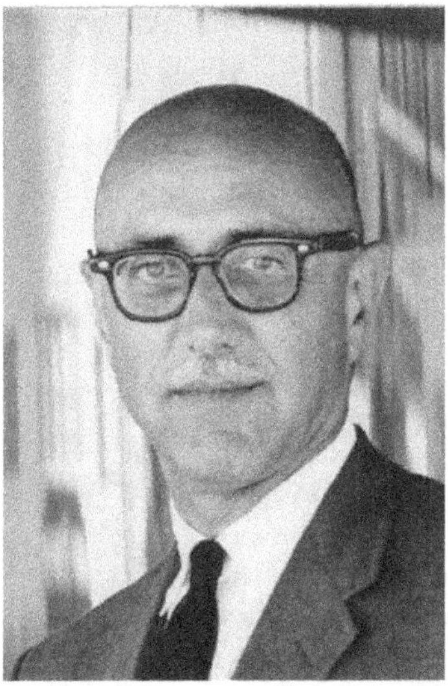

Dr. Judd Marmor has long espoused progressive views on gays and lesbians. As a well-established and highly awarded member of the psychiatric profession, he was a powerful voice in the move to depathologize homosexuality in the early 1970s. Then, as now, he has courageously held controversial positions to defend the humanity and civil rights of gays, lesbians, and others who suffer from being marginalized by society.

Dr. Marmor was born in London, England, in 1910 and emigrated with his family to Chicago in 1912. He attended Columbia University as an undergraduate and continued on to the College of Physicians and Surgeons. He undertook psychoanalytic training at the New York Psychoanalytic Institute. From 1965 to 1972, he served as Director of the Division of Psychiatry at the Cedars-Sinai Medical Center. He was the Franz Alexander Professor of Psychiatry at the University of Southern California School of Medicine from 1972 to 1980. He is now Pro-

This chapter appeared originally under the same title in *Journal of Gay & Lesbian Psychotherapy* 7(4):23-34. Copyright 2003 The Haworth Press, Inc.

doi:10.1300/6049_06

fessor Emeritus of Psychiatry at the University of California, Los Angeles.

Dr. Marmor has been a long-standing leader in psychiatry, having been President of the American Psychiatric Association, the American Academy of Psychoanalysis, the Group for the Advancement of Psychiatry, and the Southern California Psychoanalytic Society and Institute. He is a Fellow of the American College of Psychiatrists, a Founding Fellow of the American College of Psychoanalysis, and an Honorary Fellow of the Royal Australian and New Zealand College of Psychiatrists. His many awards include the Silver Medal for Distinguished Contributions to Psychiatry from the Columbia University College of Physicians and Surgeons, the Doctor of Humane Letters from Hebrew Union College, the Bowis Award from the American College of Psychiatrists, the Pawlowski Peace Prize, and the Founder's Award from the American Psychiatric Association.

Dr. Marmor has published eight books and authored or co-authored over 300 scientific articles (those related to homosexuality are listed in the concluding bibliography).

The following comments are adapted from an address Dr. Marmor gave at the University of California at Irvine in 2002, and are fol-

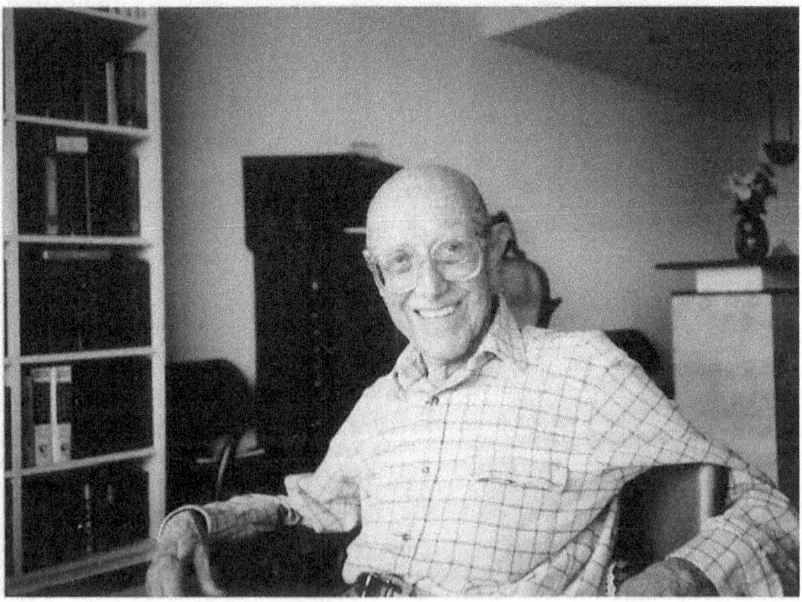

lowed by an interview conducted on July 30, 2003 in his home in Los Angeles.

While this interview was in press, Dr. Marmor passed away in Los Angeles on December 16, 2003. Obituaries marking his important contributions to the removal of homosexuality from the DSM were published in both the *Los Angeles Times* and the *New York Times*.

The American Psychiatric Association's declassification of homosexuality as a mental illness in 1973 was a bitter struggle that had a significant impact on the lives of millions of gay and lesbian women, not only in the United States but throughout the world. It was a psychiatric change that was of extraordinary sociological and psychological importance. I had the privilege of playing an important role in that decision.

Labeling homosexuality as an illness was by no means a harmless or theoretical issue. To take a position that homosexuals were inherently seriously mentally disturbed, irresponsible, and compulsively driven by needs over which they had no control had very serious social and legal consequences for them. It lent official scientific, psychiatric justification for discharging them from military service, denying them housing and other legal rights, and excluding them from various occupations and even subjecting them to arbitrary arrest and/or hospitalization.

Let me recapitulate briefly how I happened to become involved in that historic struggle.

In the early 1930s, when I graduated from medical school, the field of psychiatry was dominated by two major approaches. The older one rested on a hospital-based Kraepelinian model that viewed mental illness in terms of discrete diagnostic categories whose origins were, for the most part, attributed to genetic weaknesses, physical traumata, or infectious agents. Therapy within this model, except where a specific antidote to a noxious agent was available, was essentially nonspecific, supportive, and custodial.

At the other end of the spectrum stood the still young modality of psychoanalytic theory which postulated that most functional mental disorders could be traced to vicissitudes and conflicts in early childhood. I was among those who were strongly motivated to embrace this paradigm. Here at last seemed to be an approach that promised by rational means to enable us to unravel and thereby ameliorate the hidden sources of much human emotional distress.

Thus, in 1937, after completing the additional four years of postgraduate training in neurology and psychiatry required for certification in both of those specialties, I entered into psychoanalytic training. It was there that I first encountered the formulations of organized psychoanalytic theory concerning homosexuality. Over the next three years, as I listened to the views of my instructors about how all homosexuals were supposedly basically disturbed individuals, emotionally immature, deceptive, impulsive, unreliable, and incapable of truly loving, I found myself becoming increasingly skeptical and uneasy. It seemed to me that what I was hearing was the stereotyping and stigmatizing of an entire group of individuals, a pattern that I had already learned to distrust as a reflection of *social prejudice* in other areas, for example, toward Catholics, Jews, blacks, and other minority groups.

Then, in the late 1940s and early 1950s, I was impressed by the publication of the Kinsey group's historic studies of male and female sexuality which seemed to me to be praiseworthy efforts to study the problems of human sexuality more objectively and scientifically.[1] I also became aware in the late 1950s of Dr. Evelyn Hooker's classic studies which demonstrated that on projective tests evaluated blindly by experts, there were no demonstrable differences between a group of untreated, successful, well-adjusted homosexual men, and that of a matched group of successful, well-adjusted heterosexuals.[2]

These findings, together with my own growing conviction that causality was usually a multidimensional phenomenon and not a unidimensional one (the term "biopsychosocial" had not yet entered our vocabulary) led me in the early 1960s to put together my first book on homosexuality. The volume was called *Sexual Inversion: The Multiple Roots of Homosexuality,* and I invited contributions from experts from a wide variety of biological and social fields: history, zoology, genetics, endocrinology, sociology, and anthropology, as well as psychology and psychiatry. Because of the inadequate state of our knowledge at that time, the book had a number of limitations, as did also my later book in 1980, *Homosexual Behavior: A Modern Reappraisal,* which, although an improvement on the first, still reflected gaps in the knowledge that have since been partially filled. Nevertheless, even the first book presented some relatively fresh biosocial approaches to the issue of homosexuality. It also presented my strong affirmation that, inasmuch as the then current conclusions that psychoanalysts and psychiatrists were expressing about homosexuality were all obviously based on small samples of homosexual patients who were in treatment, it was scientifically unwarranted and biased to infer from these samples that all homosexuals were maladjusted or mentally ill. Indeed, if we were to draw our conclusions about the mental health of all heterosexuals based only on those whom we treated, we would arrive at equally unrealistic generalizations about the mental health of all heterosexuals!

More important, however, the results of that book's publication were fateful and surprising for me personally. At various subsequent psychiatric meetings and at the annual meeting of the American Psychiatric Association (APA), as well as at some of the psychoanalytic meetings, increasing numbers of reputable psychiatrists and psychoanalysts began to introduce themselves to me as being gay. I also learned for the first time of the existence of the so-called "Gay-P-A": a group of homosexual psychiatrists that met secretly during the annual meeting of the APA. They invited me to attend some of their gatherings, where I met other able colleagues like them, *all closeted in their public lives.*

As a consequence of these new experiences, the views that I had expressed in my book were strongly reinforced and I began to play an increasingly active role in meetings, debates, and panel discussions across the country, as well as in forensic legal situations. In these I attacked the prevailing psychiatric and psychoanalytic views about homosexuality and argued for its removal as a mental disorder from the APA's *Diagnostic and Statistical Manual* (DSM). I was also fortunate in being able to play an active role together with Evelyn Hooker in the work of the National Institute of Mental Health Task Force on Homosexuality between the years 1968 and 1970, and in the preparation of its progressive report that came out in 1972.

Despite my obvious involvement with the issue and probably because, as Richard Friedman[3] has tactfully put it in one of his papers, I was seen as "something of a maverick" by the existing psychoanalytic hierarchy, I was never invited to participate in the regular panel discussions and programs on homosexuality that were held under the aegis of the American Psychoanalytic Association. Nevertheless, Charles Socarides[4] and his supporters were regularly invited! It was obvious that the psychoanalytic hierarchy simply did not want to have my point of view presented.

My activity on APA programs continued at a steady rate, however, and I had the privilege of being the main psychiatric speaker at the historic meeting in 1972 at which Dr. H. Anonymous [John Fryer], the cloaked and masked gay psychiatrist, made his impressive presentation about what it meant to be a homosexual professional in a hostile culture.[5] At that meeting I again strongly condemned the existing attitudes in all the American psychoanalytic institutes in refusing to admit homosexuals for training. I also criticized the continuing pathologization of homosexuals by both psychiatry and psychoanalysis which was forcing the vast majority of them to remain closeted in self-defense. In any event, the APA's subsequent historic position statement of 1973 set off a process of progress that had important social and legal significance for the lives of homosexuals in America.

In this connection, however, I would like to comment on what has become a frequently encountered misstatement about the role that gay political pressure played in the APA's 1973 decision. This is a point that Ronald Bayer makes in his otherwise excellent volume, *Homosexuality and American Psychiatry: The Politics of Diagnosis*.[6] The fact is that the decision to remove homosexuality from the DSM was *not* based on gay political pressure but on scientific correctness, and only after a full year of exploratory hearings and study of the issue by the APA's Committee on Nomenclature, a year during which it heard presentations both by proponents and opponents of depathologization. The council was influenced by the weight of scientific studies done by Evelyn Hooker and many other psychologists by that time, as well as by reports of psychiatrists and psychoanalysts, such as Robert Stoller, Richard Green, and myself. That decision was then approved by a unanimous vote of the APA's Board of Trustees with two abstentions. The so-called "politics" surrounding the decision was subsequently instilled into the process by opponents led by Drs. Irving Bieber[7] and Charles Socarides who, because they were so outraged by the board's action, gathered names for an initiative that *forced* it to be voted on by the APA membership. That vote, to the surprise and dismay of these hard-liners, was to uphold the board's judgment.

It was regrettable that it took the American Psychoanalytic Association an additional eighteen years, until 1991, to commit itself to the enlightened views that it now officially holds.[8] Freud himself was quite open-minded on the subject of homosexuality and often remarked on the positive contributions that homosexuals make in art and civilization.[9] He also favored them being accepted for psychoanalytic training.[10] Therefore, it was paradoxical that it was this body of the self-professed disciples of Freud who continued to be recalcitrant to this new view, as indeed some of them still are!

Let me also comment briefly on Freud's occasional use of the term "perversion" in relation to homosexuality. Freud's use of the word was quite different in meaning from the sick connotation it has come to represent in our language today. He used it to refer to something that he considered to be "incorrect," but in no way sick—much as we do when we talk about something being a "perversion of the truth." Freud's use of the word was because, at that time, as an evolutionary theorist, he believed that the "correct" purpose of sex had to be a reproductive one, in the interest of species survival. Hence, what did not promote reproduction was presumably a "perversion" of sexuality. However, Freud's assumption that there is a "purpose" in natural law is no longer adhered to by most contemporary biologists, who hold that evolution proceeds without regard to either "divine" or "natural" purpose. Indeed, in today's world, uncontrolled reproduction may very well threaten the survival of mankind while, paradoxically, gay and lesbian sex tends to place desirable limits on such an unfavorable outcome.

Incidentally, you will notice that I have not used Freud's term "sexual object choice" in any of my comments. I think it is an inaccurate use of the term because it implies that homosexuality is "chosen" and that is not true. Therefore, I prefer the term "orientation" or "sexual variation" because we now know that, to a great extent, variations in sexual orientation are determined by the degree of androgenization of the fetal midbrain at a critical period of intrauterine development. We now also know that approximately 5 percent of all males, in all societies and all cultures, have a variation in the degree of prenatal androgenization that results in more or less exclusive homosexuality. Another 15 percent, approximately, have lesser degrees of androgenization that put them as partial homosexuals, from 1 to 5 on the Kinsey scale, and that is why we find a greater number of people who have tendencies toward homosexuality. However, there *are* people who are 0 (totally heterosexual) and 6 (totally homosexual) on the Kinsey scale, depending on the degree of prenatal androgenization.

In women the situation is different. Approximately 2 percent of women have a degree of androgenization that leads to a more or less biologically determined homosexuality, but women are also capable of responding to members of the same sex in a way that males who are 0 on the Kinsey scale are not. We also know that women can choose same-sex orientation for political reasons.

In time we will learn a great deal more about the biological and genetic factors of homosexual orientation, but until then we must recognize that it is not an inherent "fault." Regarding it as a flaw is a reflection of the prejudice in our culture. Again, I want to emphasize strongly that the inadequacy or inferiority that is attributed to gays and lesbians simply reflects the social prejudice of our society and does not exist in societies that treat people who are born with these differences in a much more humane, respecting, and sometimes even admiring way.

Finally, I would like to make a comment about certain ways in which we write or speak about homosexuals as if they were a special "species," instead of human beings like anyone else who just happens to have varied sexual orientations. This is just as wrong as a similar tendency to define people with different religious orientations, for example, Christians, Muslims, Jews, etc., as if they too were a separate species of mankind, instead of human beings like everyone else who happens to have been exposed to different kinds of acculturation from early childhood on.

An expression of this error is the tendency to assume that if members of such a group have a higher frequency of certain behavioral patterns, for example, depression or suicidality, that those patterns are an intrinsic aspect of that group. A flagrant example of this is the assumption that blacks, by nature, are less intelligent than whites, ignoring the profoundly different environments, both economic and cultural, in which the majority of blacks grow up in this country. Similarly, one frequently encounters statements that homosexuals or women are *inherently* more prone to depression and/or suicide, again, ignoring the influence of the hostile and prejudicial environments in which members of these groups grow up and form their identities—environments that lead them to internalize these attitudes, with consequent impairment of their self-images. It is for this reason and *not* for intrinsic ones that a greater proportion of people in these groups show a propensity toward depressive reactions and a higher incidence of suicide.

JGLP: It sounds like you have completely rejected the traditional psychoanalytic formulations of homosexuality.

DR. MARMOR: Absolutely. That was all part of Freud's reflection of the prejudices of our culture, just as his ideas about women (which I have also written extensively on) were based on the prejudices of his time.

JGLP: Why do you think the analysts were so dead set on keeping homosexuality in the DSM?

DR. MARMOR: Part of the reason was that they wanted to continue to consider it a treatable condition, and whether they realized it, consciously or not, they didn't want to let go of that for economic as well as for theoretical reasons. The continuing opposition to accepting the biological basis comes from people like Socarides who makes his living arguing that gays and lesbians are sick people, that they must be treated, and that it's an "epidemic" in our society.[11]

It's similar to the problem of anti-Semitism. All kinds of terrible things are said about people who are Jewish. But the problem is not in being Jewish; the problem is in the social prejudice of the civilization of the anti-Semite. We have to recognize that the potential of all human beings is shaped biopsychosocially and that the social, cultural, and religious influences are very powerful. When a child grows up hearing other people like him being called faggots, pansies, sissies, or worse terms, being thought of in the most ugly, demeaning ways, his image of himself becomes distorted and he develops a distorted self-image that leads to feelings of depression, neuroticism, of higher suicidality, etc. That's not inherent in being gay; it is a consequence of a civilization that creates a negative self-introject in gay people.

JGLP: What are your feelings about psychoanalysis today?

DR. MARMOR: I think many of Freud's ideas are outdated. The overemphasis on the initial triad, mother-father-child, and the failure to take into account the equally profound effects of peer group interrelationships, and of social, cultural, and religious indoctrination is a great mistake. We have made great progress in that the new views in psychiatry are biopsychosocial. But there are still carryovers, especially among analysts—and I speak as one who was trained as an analyst—to cling to Freud's ideas and reduce everything to mother, father, and child. A lot of the "interpretations" about homosexuals and the partners they choose as being based just on their attitude toward their mother and father is just sheer nonsense!

JGLP: So does psychoanalysis have a future?

DR. MARMOR: Yes, I do think psychodynamics has a future. I think it's important for us to understand that behavioral problems have a history, and for us to try to understand the biopsychosocial factors that are involved in that history, and help the patient understand them also. The future of psychoanalysis depends on the degree to which it can become less dependent on early Freudian theory and more involved with contemporary psychodynamic theory. There *is* something to be said for working intensively one-on-one with an individual; although, it doesn't have to be four or five times a week. That's baloney! But the terrible danger in today's society is that we may become so biologically and pharmacologically oriented that we may forget that there are psychodynamic factors involved, and we have to be sensitive to those factors also.

JGLP: There has been a tremendous amount of cultural change in the decades since the DSM change on homosexuality.

DR. MARMOR: We are making progress, but we still have a considerable ways to go. We still hear and read about anti-gay material. And most churches still have not changed their view. People still quote the Bible, which reflects the prejudices of earlier times, and people are still being indoctrinated with those ideas.

JGLP: The U.S. Supreme Court recently overturned anti-sodomy laws, and the Ontario Supreme Court legalized gay marriages. Marriage is the leading issue on the agenda for gay rights. Do you thing gay marriage is a good thing?

DR. MARMOR: I have always been in favor of it. I think that marriage carries with it certain rights and privileges and that gay people who want to live together should not be deprived of them. Again, it's part of the social prejudice of our time that some states are willing to call it a "civil union," but they don't want to give up the precious word "marriage." But marriage is essentially an agreement between two people to live together, to love one another, to stay together, and it carries certain privileges. I think gays and lesbians are entitled to the same thing. They are also entitled to adopt children because all the scientific evidence that we have is that gay parents have no effect on the sexual orientation of the child. So, children who are raised by gays and are loved, protected, and given warm, loving homes are getting the best of care and should not be deprived of that.

JGLP: A controversial diagnostic issue currently being debated within the APA is that of "gender identity disorder" or transsexualism. It is a somewhat similar issue to that of homosexuality in the early 1970s. What are your thoughts on the topic?

DR. MARMOR: I don't think transsexualism should be treated as a mental disorder. I think it is a genetic disorder, and it creates problems of adaptation for the transsexual, but we should not add to those problems by denigrating them as sick people. They have a different genetic factor that probably also has something to do with the degree of androgenization of the child's brain. We have to be more humane and more humanistic and treat every human being as a potentially capable and good person, unless proven otherwise. We shouldn't indoctrinate them with feelings of inferiority.

NOTES

1. See Kinsey, A., Pomeroy, W. & Martin, C. (1948), *Sexual Behavior in the Human Male*. Philadelphia, PA: Saunders; and Kinsey, A., Pomeroy, W., Martin, C. & Gebhard, P. (1953), *Sexual Behavior in the Human Female*. Philadelphia, PA: Saunders.

2. Hooker, E. (1957), The adjustment of the male overt homosexual. *J. Proj. Tech.*, 21:18-31.

3. See Friedman, R.C. & Downey, J.I. (2002), *Sexual Orientation and Psychoanalysis: Sexual Science and Clinical Practice*. New York: Columbia University Press.

4. New York psychoanalyst Charles Socarides has continued a tradition of arguing that homosexuality is a serious psychopathology that can be cured in many instances through analysis. He spearheaded the opposition to the depathologization of homosexuality in 1973. See Socarides, C.W. (1995), *Homosexuality: A Freedom Too Far*. Phoenix, AZ: Adam Margrave Books.

5. Dr. H. Anonymous was Dr. John Fryer, a Philadelphia psychiatrist who appeared on a panel at the 1973 APA meeting in disguise and spoke through a voice-distorting microphone to protect his identity. He recounts his life and this dramatic

moment in psychiatric history in David Scasta's article on John E. Fryer, MD, and the Dr. H. Anonymous episode, Chapter 1 in this book. Dr. Fryer died February 21, 2003, at the age of sixty-five.

6. See Bayer, R. (1981), *Homosexuality and American Psychiatry: The Politics of Diagnosis*. New York: Basic Books.

7. The late Irving Bieber, MD, was senior author of a landmark study of psychoanalytic efforts to convert homosexual patients to heterosexual ones. See Bieber, I., Dain, H., Dince, P., Drellich, M., Grand, H., Gundlach, R., Kremer, M., Rifkin, A., Wilbur, C. & Bieber T. (1962), *Homosexuality: A Psychoanalytic Study*. New York: Basic Books. The authors claimed a 27 percent conversion rate through psychoanalytic treatments. These results were challenged by the late C. A. Tripp, PhD, who said Bieber could not produce one successfully converted patient (see Tripp, C. A. [1975], *The Homosexual Matrix*. New York: Meridian). For the personal experience of one unsuccessfully converted patient, see Moor, P. (2001), The view from Irving Bieber's couch: "Heads I win, tails you lose." *J. of Gay & Lesbian Psychotherapy*, 5(3/4):25-36. Reprinted in: *Sexual Conversion Therapy: Ethical, Clinical and Research Perspectives*, ed. A. Shidlo, M. Schroeder & J. Drescher. Binghamton, NY: The Haworth Press, 2001, pp. 25-36.

8. See Roughton, R. (1995), Overcoming antihomosexual bias: A progress report. *The American Psychoanalyst*, 29(4):15-16.

9. See Freud, S. (1905), Three essays on the theory of sexuality. *Standard Edition*, 7:123-246. London: Hogarth Press, 1953; and Freud, S. (1935), Anonymous (Letter to an American mother). In: *The Letters of Sigmund Freud*, ed. E. Freud. New York: Basic Books, 1960, pp. 423-424.

10. Editor's Note: In the 1970s, a letter was found in the Columbia University archives. This "Circular Letter" was written by Freud and Otto Rank in 1921 to Freud's inner circle in response to another member of that circle, Ernest Jones, who opposed admitting any homosexual candidates for psychoanalytic training. Freud disagreed and said, "We feel that a decision in such cases should depend upon a thorough examination of the [candidate's] other qualities." The letter was first published by an early Canadian gay rights organization in *Body Politic* (Toronto), May 1977, p. 9. It was reprinted in Lewes, K. (1988), *The Psychoanalytic Theory of Male Homosexuality*. New York: Simon and Schuster, p. 33.

11. See Marmor, J. (1970), "Homosexuality and objectivity." *SIECUS Newsletter*, 6(2):1, 3.

SELECTED BIBLIOGRAPHY

Books

Seward, G.H. (1956), *Psychotherapy and Culture Conflict, with Case Studies by Judd Marmor*. New York: Ronald Press.

Group for the Advancement of Psychiatry (GAP) (1964), *Psychiatric Aspects of the Prevention of Nuclear War, Formulated by the Committee on Social Issues*, ed. J. Marmor (GAP Report no. 57). New York: GAP.

Marmor, J. (1965), *Sexual Inversion: The Multiple Roots of Homosexuality.* New York: Basic Books.

Marmor, J., ed. (1968), *Modern Psychoanalysis: New Directions and Perspectives.* New York: Basic Books.

Marmor, J. (1974), *Psychiatry in Transition: Selected Papers.* New York: Brunner/Mazel.

Marmor, J. (1975), *Psychiatrists and Their Patients: A National Study of Private Office Practice.* Washington, DC: American Psychiatric Association and the National Association for Mental Health.

Marmor, J. (1980), *Homosexual Behavior: A Modern Reappraisal.* New York: Basic Books.

Marmor, J. & Woods, S.M., eds. (1980), *The Interface Between the Psychodynamic and Behavioral Therapies.* New York: Plenum Medical Book.

Eisenstein, S., Levy, N.A. & Marmor, J. (1994), *The Dyadic Transaction: An Investigation into the Nature of the Psychotherapeutic Process.* New Brunswick, NJ: Transaction Publishers.

Nardi, P.M., Sanders, D. & Marmor, J., eds. (1994), *Growing Up Before Stonewall: Life Stories of Some Gay Men.* New York: Routledge.

Marmor, J. (1994), *Psychiatry in Transition,* Second Edition. New Brunswick, NJ: Transaction Publishers.

Marmor, J. (1995), *Modern Psychoanalysis: New Directions and Perspectives,* Second Edition. New Brunswick, NJ: Transaction Publishers.

Selected Articles and Book Chapters

Marmor, J. (1958), Changing patterns of sexual identity. In: *Current Trends in Psychiatry.* Des Plaines, IL: Forest Hospital Foundation, pp. 138-309.

Marmor, J. (1964), Understanding the homosexual patient. (An interview by Marijo Juzwiak.) *RN Magazine,* 27:53-59.

Marmor, J. (1967), Changing feminine gender role (Abstract). *Newsletter of the Southern California Psychiatric Society,* 14(1):6.

Marmor, J. (1967), Le problème de l'homosexualité vue d'ensemble. *Médecine et hygiene,* 788:371.

Marmor, J. (1970), Homosexuality and objectivity. *SIECUS Newsletter,* 6(2):1, 3.

Marmor, J. (1971), Discussion of article by Jules Bemporad, "An attempt to define sexual deviation." *The [American Academy of Psychoanalysis] Forum* 1(2):4.

Marmor, J. (1971), Homosexuality in males. *Psychiatr. Ann.,* 1:44-59.

Marmor, J. (1971), "Normal" and "deviant" sexual behavior. *J. Am. Med. Assn.,* 217:165-170.

Marmor, J. (1972), Homosexuality—Mental illness or moral dilemma? *Int. J. Psychiat.,* 10:114-117.

Marmor, J. (1972), Notes on some psychodynamic aspects of homosexuality. In: *National Institute of Mental Health Task Force on Homosexuality: Final Report and Background Papers,* ed. John M. Livingood. DHEW publication no. (ADM)

76-357. Rockville, MD: U.S. Department of Health, Education, and Welfare, pp. 55-57.

Marmor, J. (1972), Psychotherapy of homosexuals. *Medical Aspects of Human Sexuality* (Oct.):137-138.

Marmor, J. (1973), Homosexuality and cultural value systems. *Am. J. Psychiat.*, 131:780.

Marmor, J. (1973), Is homosexuality pathologic or a normal variant of sexuality? *Medical Aspects of Human Sexuality* (Dec.):10-15.

Marmor, J. (1974), Homosexuality. In: *Sexuality and Human Values,* ed. M. Calderone. New York: Association Press, pp. 23-33.

Marmor, J. (1975), Homosexuality and sexual orientation disturbances. In: *Comprehensive Textbook of Psychiatry,* Second Edition, ed. H. Kaplan & A. Freedman. Baltimore, MD: Williams & Wilkins, pp. 1510-1520.

Marmor, J. (1976), Homosexuality and sexual orientation disturbances. In: *The Sexual Experience,* ed. B. Sadock, H. Kaplan & A. Freedman. Baltimore, MD: Williams & Wilkins, pp. 374-391.

Marmor, J. (1976), Homosexuality in twins. *Medical Aspects of Human Sexuality* (Apr.):72-73.

Marmor, J. & Green, R. (1977), Homosexuality. In: *Handbook of Sexology,* ed. J. Money & H. Musaph. Amsterdam: Elsevier, pp. 1051-1068.

Marmor, J. (1977), Homosexuality: An overview. In: *International Encyclopedia of Psychiatry, Psychology, Psychoanalysis, and Neurology,* ed. B.B. Wolman. New York: Aesculapius Press, Volume 5, pp. 407-410.

Marmor, J. (1985), Homosexuality: Nature vs. nurture. *Harvard Medical School Mental Health Letter,* 2(4).

Chapter 6

An Interview with Robert L. Spitzer, MD

Jack Drescher

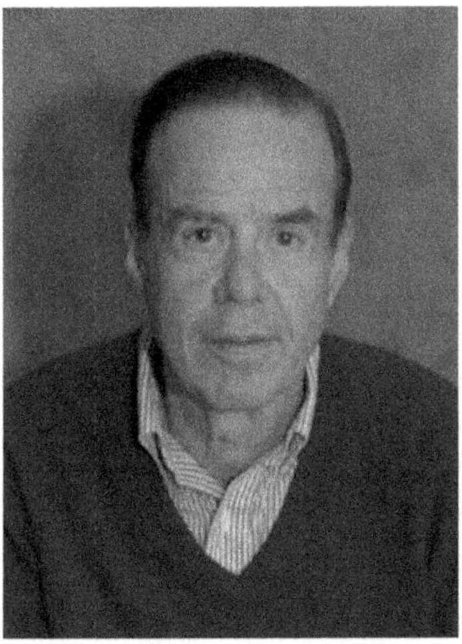

The *Journal of Gay & Lesbian Psychotherapy* has been publishing a series of biographical interviews of psychiatrists and other mental health professionals who have made important contributions to psychiatric attitudes about gay and lesbian patients and toward enhancing the lives of gay and lesbian therapists. Robert L. Spitzer, MD, has had a profound impact on both groups. As a junior member of the American Psychiatric Association's (APA) Committee on Nomenclature, Dr. Spitzer helped shepherd a process that led to the 1973 removal of the diagnosis of homosexuality from the *Diagnostic and Statistical Manual* (DSM).

Dr. Spitzer is Professor of Psychiatry, Columbia University, and Chief of the Biometrics Research Department at the New York State Psychiatric Institute. He has achieved national and international recognition as an authority in psychiatric assessment and the classification of mental disorders. He is the author of over 280 articles on psychiatric assessment and diagnosis.

This chapter appeared originally under the same title in *Journal of Gay & Lesbian Psychotherapy* 7(3):97-111.

American Psychiatry and Homosexuality: An Oral History
Published by The Haworth Press, Inc., 2007.
doi:10.1300/6049_07

In 1974, the American Psychiatric Association appointed Dr. Spitzer to chair its Committee on Nomenclature and Statistics, and in this capacity he assumed the leadership role in the development of DSM-III,[1] published in 1980, which became the authoritative classification of mental disorders for the mental health professions, not only in this country, but internationally.

In 1983, Dr. Spitzer was appointed to chair the American Psychiatric Association's Work Group to Revise DSM-III and coordinated that effort, resulting in the publication of DSM-III-R[2] in the spring of 1987. He was active in the development of DSM-IV,[3] as a special advisor to the American Psychiatric Association's Task Force on DSM-IV.

Dr. Spitzer has received numerous honors from his professional colleagues. Among these are the American Psychiatric Association's 1987 Adolf Meyer Award for "outstanding contributions to the science and practice of psychiatry." In 1994, he received the American Psychiatric Association's Award for Psychiatric Research for his contributions to psychiatric assessment and diagnosis. In 2000, he was the Thomas William Salmon Medal recipient from the New York Academy of Medicine for "outstanding contributions to psychiatry."

Dr. Spitzer has pioneered in the development of several widely used diagnostic assessment procedures, including the Research Diagnostic Criteria, the Schedule for Affective Disorders and Schizophrenia (SADS), and the Structured Clinical Interview for DSM-IV (SCID). His most recent research efforts have been in the development of the PRIME-MD, a widely used instrument designed to assist physicians and researchers in the recognition and diagnosis of mental disorders in the primary care setting.

JGLP: Where are you from and how did you decide to become a psychiatrist?

DR. SPITZER: I grew up in Manhattan. Actually I was born in White Plains, lived in Scarsdale till I was two, then lived in Manhattan until I went to college at Cornell. I grew up in the 1930s and 1940s and my mother was a big fan of psychoanalysis. She was kind of a chronic outpatient in psychoanalysis. In fact, one of her therapists was Judd Marmor before he moved from New York to Los Angeles.[4] In fact, when I used to meet Judd Marmor every now and then at the APA annual meetings he used to ask, "How is your mom doing?"

So the idea of becoming a psychoanalyst seemed naturally what I wanted to do. I went to medical school for that reason. There was a very brief period when I was thinking of internal medicine, but I pretty much always wanted to be a psychiatrist, and specifically a psychoanalyst. I was a psychology major at Cornell and then went to NYU School of Medicine. I did an internship at Montefiore Hospital where they allowed you to take a four- to six-week elective elsewhere, and I took one at the Psychiatric Institute (PI). I think because of that, and because I had published some articles as a medical student I was accepted into PI as a resident in 1958 and I've really been there ever since. No one's offered me a good job so I've stayed there *[laughs]*. So that's how I got into psychiatry.

JGLP: When you decided you were going to be a psychiatrist and were getting your psychiatric training, who were the people most influential in the development of your own thinking as a psychiatrist and a psychoanalyst?

DR. SPITZER: I was in my second year of residency at Columbia when I became a student at the Columbia Psychoanalytic Center—they've changed the name since then.[5] I started off with Abraham Kardiner as my analyst.[6] I chose him because I felt I needed somebody really experienced if I was going to make any fundamental change. That didn't work out, so I switched to Arnold Cooper, who was, at the time, very influential in my thinking. He had been a supervisor of mine and I saw that he had a very different approach to treating patients than all of my other analytic teachers. Another person who was influential was Will Gaylin. Those were the big teachers for me at the time. Rado had just about finished when I came there. Rado was no longer the director of the center when I came there.[7]

JGLP: You didn't have any contact with him.

DR. SPITZER: I didn't. I think he gave one or two lectures, but he was pretty much finished.

JGLP: Did you finish your analytic training?

DR. SPITZER: I actually graduated—barely—from the Columbia Psychoanalytic Center.

JGLP: How is that you came to pursue research rather than a career in psychoanalysis?

DR. SPITZER: When I started my residency, my thought was I would do both clinical work and research. The research that interested me was evaluation of treatment. That was what really turned me on. The nice thing about Psychiatric Institute in those days was that they had a lunch room where the staff and the residents ate with the senior research people. They even had nice tables with linen and silverware. There, I became friendly with Joe Zubin, who was head of the Biometrics Research Department. When I finished my residency, I started a fellowship with him, and that got me into rating scales and standardized interview schedules.

But at that time I wasn't that interested in diagnosis, so I got into diagnosis—again, by whom I met at lunch. One of the people who had lunch at PI was Ernie Gruenberg, a well-known psychiatric epidemiologist. This was 1968 and I had been a research fellow in Joe Zubin's Biometric Research Department for a few years. One day at lunch Gruenberg said, "I'm chairing a committee that's developing DSM-II.[8] We're almost done. I could use somebody who could take notes and maybe do a little editing. Would you be interested?" I said, "Is there any money involved?" He said, "No." I made a quick decision. I said, "Well, that's not important." As a result of that, I joined his committee and helped edit DSM-II. There's a little introduction to DSM-II that I wrote. So that's how I got into the APA, DSM business.

Then, when DSM-II was finished, the Committee on Nomenclature kept meeting. They have not been meeting between editions since DSM-III. But in those days, between the first and second editions, there was always a Committee on Nomenclature that would meet once or twice a year. They wouldn't have very much to do, but they would meet. What they mainly did was answer letters from record room librarians asking things like, "How do I code mental retardation with psychosis?" So I joined the committee after DSM-II was completed in 1968. A few years later, I became involved in the homosexuality controversy and that's how I became known to people like Judd Marmor. As a result, in 1974, I was appointed to chair the committee that developed DSM-III.

JGLP: What happened around the homosexuality controversy?

DR. SPITZER: Well, first off, pretty much everybody who was trained in those years took it for granted that homosexuality was not only an illness, but it was a very severe illness. It was considered not just an illness of sexual functioning, but really a widespread personality disturbance. The psychoanalysts at Columbia had a special interest in this area because of Rado, I guess, and some of the people there had written several articles on the treatment of homosexuality. Lionel Ovesey had written about the treatment of homosexuality and also taught that homosexuality had to be distinguished from pseudohomosexuality—the fear that a passive heterosexual might have of being homosexual.[9] So that was the way I saw things as well.

Then, I guess it was around 1972, I was becoming disenchanted with psychoanalysis. I did some clinical work as an analyst, but I never really felt very comfortable doing it. I became interested in a lot of different kinds of nonanalytic psychotherapy. At that time, I was very interested in behavior therapy. There was a meeting of the Association for the Advancement of Behavior Therapy, and they had a symposium on the treatment of homosexuality. They had invited some poor guy from London to come all the way to New York to give a talk. So I'm at this symposium and about ten minutes into it, a group of gay activists[10] started standing up. I don't remember exactly what they said, but essentially what they said was, "This meeting has got to stop! We can't take this anymore. You're pathologizing us!" The chair of the symposium tried to get them to stop, but eventually said, "Okay, the meeting is over." The poor guy from London never got to present his stuff *[chuckles]*.

I felt this was pretty awful, breaking up a meeting. I went over to one of the guys demonstrating, Ron Gold, and I introduced myself. It turned out we actually had a friend in common, but I didn't know it at the time. I told him I really thought that it was pretty awful, breaking up the meeting. We got to talking and somehow it came out that I was on this APA Committee on Nomenclature and Statistics. He said, "Gee, could my group talk to your group?" So I thought, "Gee, that's an interesting idea." So I went back to the committee. The chairman of that committee was Henry Brill, a state hospital administrator. I said there's this group that would like to meet with us. Of course, at this time there was a lot of furor in psychiatry. Gays were saying how terrible things were being done to them by psychiatry pathologizing homosexuality. It was not a new idea that there was some controversy.[11] Brill said, "Okay, let's meet with them and see what happens." We arranged for this meeting; I'm not sure how many of them came. I was talking to Charles Silverstein who remembers it better than I do, since he was at the meeting.[12]

So this group came and gave their presentation, where they essentially said there's no scientific basis for this diagnosis; that terrible things are done to homosexuals. I'm not sure if they said it explicitly, but implicit was the idea that the only way gays could overcome civil rights discrimination was if psychiatry would acknowledge that homosexuality was not a mental illness. So they left the meeting. I don't know how they felt their presentation went over, but when they left Brill turned to me and he said, "Okay, Bob, you've gotten us into this mess. Now what do we do?" So I came up with the idea of, "Let's have a symposium." I organized a symposium at that year's APA 1973 annual meeting which was held in Hawaii. If I remember correctly who was on the symposium, it was Robert Stoller, Richard Green, Judd Marmor, Ron Gold, Irving Bieber, and Charles Socarides.[13]

During the several months before this symposium, I started having more contact with Ron Gold and other colleagues of his. It was really the first time that I had any personal contact with people—although I'm sure I had had contact without knowing it—that were openly homosexual. It was quite a different experience for me because they became human people. I started to think, "What could be done with this?" I guess my own feelings were of compassion, wanting to be helpful. At the same time, wanting to do what made sense scientifically. So my own view started to change in terms of basic assumptions. Now, how much of that was a result of true scientific logic? I would like to think that part of it was that. But certainly a large part of it was just feeling that they were right! That if they were going to be successful in overcoming discrimination, this clearly was something that had to change.

I started to think, "Was there some way to resolve what seemed like totally incompatible viewpoints?" On the one hand, there was the traditional view that homosexuality was an illness, a serious illness, which should be treated.[14] On the other hand, there was the argument that it was just normal variation. I like to think that later, when I was working on DSM-III, that I was very good at a kind of nosological diplomacy, in other words, thinking of compromises that could move and resolve a controversy. I started to think, "Okay, psychiatry has never defined mental disorder," and that was now clearly the issue. Of course, in general medicine, there is no accepted definition, but general medicine doesn't really feel a need to have one. But clearly if you're going to have some people saying homosexuality is not a mental disorder, well, then what is a mental disorder?

To answer that question, I said to myself, "Well, why don't you look through DSM-II, look at all the different disorders, and ask yourself is there something that intuitively stands out—something that all these diagnoses share?" As I did that, of course, I'm thinking in the back of my mind, "Is there something that they all share that I can argue does not apply to homosexuality?" Well, what they seemed to by and large all share was that people who had these conditions were usually not very happy about it. They had distress, or if they didn't have distress, in some way the condition interfered with their overall functioning. What was clear was that, where it used to be thought that every homosexual must be dissatisfied with their condition, if you accepted what the activists said, clearly there were homosexuals who were not distressed by being homosexual. Instead, they might be distressed by how people reacted to their being gay.

I concluded that the solution was to argue that a mental disorder must be associated with either distress or general impairment. The reason I said "general" was that you could certainly argue that homosexuals can't function heterosexually. Of course, the gays say, "Well, heterosexuals can't function homosexually." So I said "Well, it's not just functioning; it's generalized functioning," and that was around the time when there were several studies showing that if you compared general psychopathology among non-patient gays in the community and nongays, there weren't many differences. There was also Hooker's study showing no difference in terms of at least obvious psychopathology.[15]

So based on that, one could argue, Yes, there were some new scientific findings about homosexuals and here's a definition of mental disorder that makes some sense; and based on that, homosexuality should not be in the DSM-II.

When DSM-II came out in 1968, there was no talk of DSM-III. In 1973, what we were actually talking about was successive printings of DSM-II. Every time they would run out of copies, they would print enough to last another six months or so. The issue really was, "Should the next printing of DSM-II have homosexuality in it?" As I assessed the political situation, there was no way that the membership or the APA was going to stand for totally removing the category.

There was also the whole issue of, "Can you treat homosexuality? Should you? Is it effective?" I believed in my own mind, that although homosexuality might not be an illness or a mental disorder, if somebody with homosexuality wanted to be treated, there ought to be a way of giving that person some kind of a diagnostic label. I came up with the idea of "sexual orientation disturbance."[16] Part of that was political; I knew that there was no way that homosexuality was going to be removed entirely from DSM-II, but if you had a category where you could say, "Okay, for the homosexual who's dissatisfied, you can still treat it and that's the disorder—sexual orientation disturbance." With that proposal, the Committee on Nomenclature, this small little group, approved removing homosexuality and replacing it with sexual orientation disturbance. The proposal[17] went through several other steps: the Council on Research and Development, to whom our committee answered, the APA Assembly of District Branches, and finally the Reference Committee. That committee[18] sent it along to the board of trustees and they voted on it.[19] I don't recall whether it was unanimous, but I think it may have been.[20]

In any case it was approved. Then, as many people know, the group that opposed this included Socarides, Bieber, and colleagues. They organized a petition because, at that time, the constitution of the APA had a provision where if they could get 200 members to sign this petition, you could vote on anything you wanted. They subsequently changed that bylaw *[laughs];* they don't want that to happen again. So this group initiated a referendum to undo the decision of the board of trustees. There was a several-month period during which there was heated debate and letters going out, and I became kind of the ring leader of the group, arguing not to allow this referendum to overturn the decision. I worked with the gay group and at one point we had a mailing that went out which they helped fund. The membership voted, and I think it was something like 60 percent in support to 40 percent opposed.[21] Now I'm sure that had the vote been homosexuality in or out, with no compromise category, there was no way that would have passed. So in retrospect, I think that my strategy was very successful.

Now, what I think I have to say is how do I now feel about two things: there's both the decision and the logic of the definition of mental disorder. First of all, as far as the definition of mental disorder, I've given that a lot of thought over the last thirty years. A lot of other people have given it thought, and I would certainly not defend my 1973 definition now because I think it's quite inadequate. Its inadequacies were actually pointed out at the time by the group opposed to removing homosexuality from DSM-II. Bieber said, "Well, what does that mean—you're going to throw out all the paraphilias?" Because certainly some of them are not necessarily associated with distress or impairment. At the time, I really had no answer to that. In fact there was a debate that I had with Bieber that was published in the *New York Times*.[22] It came out just a few days after the 1973 decision. We debated the definition. I must say in retrospect, I think that I would have difficulty with some of his arguments at the present time. Because, for example, recently there's been a move to change the criteria for pedophilia on the grounds that if it does not cause distress or general impairment in functioning, it's not a disorder. Well, I think pedophilia is a disorder whether it distresses you or not. So in terms of the 1973 definition I wouldn't defend it, but I think there's nothing wrong with thinking, thirty years later, that things are a little more complicated than you had originally thought. As far as the 1973 decision itself, I certainly think more people have been helped than have been hurt. I'm proud that I had something to do with it.

JGLP: Fast-forward to recent events where you find yourself once again in a controversy surrounding homosexuality.

DR. SPITZER: *[Laughs]* What recent events?

JGLP: How did you get interested in the issue of sexual conversion or, as you call it, "sexual reorientation" therapy?

DR. SPITZER: It's funny, because in some ways there are interesting parallels. I got into the original 1973 controversy because I was at this meeting where I started to talk to the people breaking up a meeting. In 1999, there was a protest at the APA annual meeting by some ex-gay groups. I don't know exactly which groups, but essentially the religious ex-gay groups. They may have had about thirty or forty people marching in front of the convention center with signs saying things like, "Homosexuality can be changed. APA is doing terrible things by declassifying it." I started to talk to one of these guys, and he tried to tell me about how he had changed. And, I admit, there is something in me that is always looking for trouble or something to challenge the orthodoxy. After talking to him—and he just talked about himself; I don't remember exactly what he said—I got the idea, "Gee, could it really be that maybe there are some gays that can change?" Now what did I think thirty years ago about treating homosexuality? I'm trying to recall what was my attitude about the possibility of change? There's one actual fact that says something about my attitude back then. It was probably in the late 1970s or early 1980s. Geraldo Rivera did a television show on whether gays can go straight. I remember Socarides was there. The television producer had called up the American Psychiatric Association. He asked, who could they suggest that would answer Socarides? I was the natural choice. I remember being on this program. Socarides brought a few of his former patients, and there were also some religious ex-gays. I gave the American Psychiatric line, which was that there were only anecdotal reports of change, no real case studies, and it was probably very unlikely that anybody could change.

Anyway, back to 1999. I got the idea, "Gee, well maybe it's not so open and shut about changing sexual orientation." Certainly, the conventional wisdom for many years was that gays could change their behavior, but they're not going to actually change their feelings. That all the gays who claim to change, what they've really changed is how they see themselves. Well, this guy and others claimed that real change of feelings was possible. So I got the idea, "How about having a debate on this?" So I proposed a symposium with myself as chair and with two people on either side.

About six weeks before the symposium was to happen, the gay side withdrew. Marshall Forstein,[23] who was going to be in the debate, wrote me that he decided not to participate. A few months before the symposium started, it occurred to me that what everybody was going to say was that we don't really have the data to answer the question about the possibility of changing sexual orientation. So I got the idea, "Maybe I could actually do a study." So Forstein wrote, "I'm not participating, both because NARTH[24] is using it politically, and also because you clearly cannot be an impartial moderator." So I wrote him back and I said, "No problem about me being a moderator; we can find somebody else. The Scientific Program Committee can find somebody else." I don't recall if he answered me; I think he did. So I spoke to the chairperson of the Scientific Program Committee, Rodrigo Muñoz, and I said, "Listen, these guys have withdrawn from the debate. That's not fair—you should let the other side present." And he essentially said, "Bob, how can you do this to your career? You must be crazy to do this." He wasn't going to help me, so the debate never happened. NARTH, of course, picketed. They had a press conference at which I appeared. For them I was the big cheese there.

JGLP: They ran a full-page ad in *USA Today* attacking the APA.

DR. SPITZER: Yes, and Dr. Laura[25] mentioned "the debate that never was" and she said, "Who do you think withdrew from the debate?" So that's that. So I decided to do this study. I've done it and that's all history.

JGLP: There was not only the issue of the canceled 2000 debate, but also what happened when you presented your preliminary findings in New Orleans the following year at the 2001 APA annual meeting. That drew a lot of media attention.[26] How do you feel doing this study has affected your professional career? How have you been personally affected by the experience?

DR. SPITZER: That's a tough question. I'm glad I did the study. I'm not entirely satisfied with the way I wrote it up and, as you know, I'm now deciding on how to respond to the twenty-five commentators on the study that will appear in the *Archives of Sexual Behavior*.[27] I think the study had value. I try to think, "Why wasn't I able to take a more measured approach?" I think part of it was the study so quickly became politicized. When I first started the study, without really having any data, there was such rage at me from gay colleagues that I think it stiffened my back, which was unfortunate. I got a lot of hate mail. But my career? You know, I'm seventy. I've had a distinguished career *[laughs]*. I mean, people still talk to me. You talk to me; we have lunch together. I regret that I didn't write it up in a more measured way.

JGLP: Is there anything you would say, in a calm moment, without your back up against the wall, to those who would say you have given aid and comfort to the enemy?

DR. SPITZER: Well, there is no doubt about that. I think there's an interesting—what is it, ethical, philosophical?—issue. I have given aid and comfort to the enemy. I suppose more people were hurt than might be helped, but I believe the study had some scientific value. What do you do in such a case? I think the study does provide some information that is of value which was not there before the study. I think that as a scientist you are entitled to study what you decide is of scientific interest. Also, you never know how many people you're going to hurt or not.

Now one of the main concerns was that the Christian Right is going to use the study to argue, "Okay, this shows that gays can change. Therefore, homosexuality is really a choice. Therefore, they're not entitled to 'special rights.'" I've been interested in how the Christian Right has used this study, and you and I have had this discussion before. In the case of Finland,[28] there was clearly the use of the study to directly say, "We should not legitimize gay civil unions." So there I did the best I could to not let my study be used in that way, and you helped with that. I appreciate that. As far as I can see, I don't see evidence of the same thing happening in America. In other words, in legal issues like the sodomy laws, I don't think the Christian Right, to my knowledge, and I think I would know about it, have used the study to support their political agenda. Now, have they used it in a general sense to support their viewpoint? Have they said, "Spitzer, who has some credibility, has shown that gays can change?" Sure they have! There's no doubt about that. But in the more specific use of saying, "Okay, this shows a direct connection; gays can change, so therefore they should not be given the rights they are asking for," I don't think they've done that.

JGLP: And on the other side, what would you say to people on the conservative religious Right?

DR. SPITZER: Well, it's kind of funny. They take pleasure in saying, "Spitzer is for gay marriage, he's for gays in the military, so he can't be accused of bias." I mean, they kind of take pleasure in that.

JGLP: So what would your response to them be?

DR. SPITZER: As far as I can see, except for the Finland [case], I don't see how they have used my study. I'm not going to say, "You should never mention Spitzer's study."

JGLP: What would you say to them in reference to fighting gay and lesbian civil rights protection?

DR. SPITZER: I've made it very clear to them that I support all those things, gays in the military, and civil unions. You know, in my article about my study, one of the things I've been accused of is dismissing the issue of harm. I don't think that's fair. I think in the article it acknowledges there is concern about harm. But that's not what my study is about.

JGLP: What are you working on now?

DR. SPITZER: *[Laughs]* I suppose I'm working on overcoming my block on writing my response to the twenty-five commentaries on my study. *[Laughs]* Of those, the majority are very critical and about ten say, "Unethical, should not be published." "Spitzer has given up scientific objectivity," you know. This is painful. One of the contributors, Milton Wainberg, his article has, I don't know, twenty co-authors.[29] I guess his point is, well, what is his point? It's like a petition to denounce me. That's okay.

JGLP: Are you working on any other research projects?

DR. SPITZER: Other research? There is life after this? I'm doing a study of dimensional systems for personality assessment because there's a lot of dissatisfaction with the traditional categorical approach to personality diagnosis. Psychologists for years have been saying that dimensional systems make more sense, but no one has actually done a study to see whether clinicians using dimensional find it more useful. I'm in the middle of that study, and that's kind of fun There's a DSM casebook that has come out for each edition: DSM-III, DSM-R, DSM-IV. There's now going to be a companion casebook where we have big-shot clinicians who will write on how they would approach the treatment of thrity-five different diagnoses.

JGLP: And you're going to be a discussant on a panel at the 2003 APA in San Francisco where the presenters argue to remove some other DSM diagnoses.

DR. SPITZER: *[Chuckles]* Paraphilias and GID [gender identity disorder]. It's interesting because the argument about homosexuality is the opening wedge. Their argument is that if homosexuality is not a disorder, why should anything connected with sex be a disorder? I have to come up with some good reasons for retaining these diagnoses. The issue is social constructionism versus essentialism. There's the appeal. These people—transgender, transsexual—all these people who have been treated terribly, just the way the gays have. So if you have any sympathy for these people, "Let's get these diagnoses out of this bloody book." This argument has some intuitive appeal. I was thinking of starting off my discussion by asking the audience to vote on how many of them agree, before they heard me, with the previous speakers. I think that most of the people in that audience will be sympathetic to those speakers arguing for removing these diagnoses from the DSM.

NOTES

1. American Psychiatric Association (1980), *Diagnostic and Statistical Manual of Mental Disorders,* Third Edition. Washington, DC: American Psychiatric Press.

2. American Psychiatric Association (1987), *Diagnostic and Statistical Manual of Mental Disorders,* Third Edition–Revised. Washington, DC: American Psychiatric Press.

3. American Psychiatric Association (1994), *Diagnostic and Statistical Manual of Mental Disorders,* Fourth Edition. Washington, DC: American Psychiatric Press.

4. Judd Marmor, MD, a member of the *JGLP*'s editorial board, is a past president of the American Psychiatric Association. In addition to his early scholarly work on nonpathological psychiatric theorizing about homosexuality (see Marmor, J., ed. [1965], *Sexual Inversion: The Multiple Roots of Homosexuality.* New York: Basic Books), Dr. Marmor was also a key figure in the removal of homosexuality from the DSM (see Bayer, R. [1981], *Homosexuality and American Psychiatry: The Politics of Diagnosis.* New York: Basic Books).

5. It is now known as the Columbia University Center for Psychoanalytic Training and Research.

6. Kardiner, A. (1955), *Sex and Morality.* London: Routledge and Kegan Paul LTD.

7. Sandor Rado was the founder of the Columbia Institute (see Roazen, P. & Swerdloff, B. [1995], *Heresy: Sandor Rado and the Psychoanalytic Movement.* Northvale, NJ: Aronson) and a major figure in post-Freudian theorizing about homosexuality and its characterization as psychopathology (see Rado, S. [1940], A critical examination of the concept of bisexuality. *Psychosomatic Med.,* 2:459-467. Reprinted in: *Sexual Inversion: The Multiple Roots of Homosexuality,* ed. J. Marmor. New York: Basic Books, 1965, pp. 175-189; and Rado, S. [1969], *Adaptational Psychodynamics: Motivation and Control.* New York: Science House).

8. American Psychiatric Association (1968), *Diagnostic and Statistical Manual of Mental Disorders,* Second Edition. Washington, DC: American Psychiatric Press.

9. Ovesey, L. (1969), *Homosexuality and Pseudohomosexuality.* New York: Science House.

10. The Gay Activists Alliance, see Bayer, *Homosexuality and American Psychiatry,* p. 115.

11. See David Scasta's article on John E. Fryer, MD, and the Dr. H. Anonymous episode, Chapter 1 in this book.

12. Charles Silverstein, PhD, is a member of the editorial board of the *Journal of Gay & Lesbian Psychotherapy.* His account of that meeting, "Are You Saying That Homosexuality Is Normal?," excerpted from his forthcoming book *For the Ferryman,* will appear in a future issue of the *JGLP.* Also see Bayer, *Homosexuality and American Psychiatry,* pp. 117-121.

13. Bayer, *Homosexuality and American Psychiatry,* p. 125.

14. Bieber, I., Dain, H., Dince, P., Drellich, M., Grand, H., Gundlach, R., Kremer, M., Rifkin, A., Wilbur, C. & Bieber, T. (1962), *Homosexuality: A Psychoanalytic Study.* New York: Basic Books; Hatterer, L. (1970), *Changing Homosexuality in the Male.* New York: McGraw Hill; and Socarides, C. (1968), *The Overt Homosexual.* New York: Grune & Stratton.

15. Hooker, E. (1957), The adjustment of the male overt homosexual. *J. Proj. Tech.,* 21:18-31.

16. According to sexual orientation disturbance (SOD) criteria, only those who were "bothered by," "in conflict with," or "wished to change" their homosexuality had a mental disorder. SOD, however, had two significant conceptual problems. First, the diagnosis could also apply to heterosexuals, a solution to APA's internal debate that did not quite concur with clinical reality. There were no reported cases of unhappy heterosexual individuals seeking psychiatric treatment to become gay or lesbian. This overinclusiveness was resolved in the DSM-III where SOD was in turn replaced by ego-dystonic homosexuality (EDH). The name change, however, did not resolve a thornier conceptual issue, which was that of making patients' subjective experiences of their own homosexuality *the determining factor* of their illness. To rely upon patient subjectivity alone was now incongruous with the new evidence-based approach that psychiatry was embracing. This ultimately led, in 1987, to EDH being removed from the DSM-III-R.

17. Spitzer, R.L. (1973), A proposal about homosexuality and the APA nomenclature: Homosexuality as an irregular form of sexual behavior and sexual orientation disturbance as a psychiatric disorder. A symposium: Should homosexuality be in the APA nomenclature? *Amer. J. Psychiatry,* 130:1207-1216.

18. The Reference Committee was comprised of the chairs of the various APA councils and the president-elect of the APA (Bayer, *Homosexuality and American Psychiatry,* p. 134).

19. December 15, 1973 (Bayer, *Homosexuality and American Psychiatry,* p. 135).

20. There were eighteen APA trustees at the time, three of whom were absent for the vote. At the final vote, thirteen voted to remove homosexuality and replace it with sexual orientation disturbance; none opposed, and two abstained (Bayer, *Homosexuality and American Psychiatry,* p. 137).

21. Of 10,091 psychiatrists voting, 58 percent voted in support of the board of trustees, 37 percent opposed the board's decision, and 3 percent abstained (Bayer, *Homosexuality and American Psychiatry,* p. 148).

22. *The New York Times,* Sunday, December 23, 1973.

23. Marshall Forstein, MD, is a past president of the Association of Gay and Lesbian Psychiatrists and a member of the editorial board of the *Journal of Gay & Lesbian Psychotherapy.*

24. The National Association for Research and Therapy of Homosexuality (NARTH), whose founders include Charles Socarides and Joseph Nicolosi. "NARTH's primary goal is to make effective psychological therapy available to all homosexual men and women who seek change" (http://narth.com/menus/goals.html).

25. Conservative commentator Dr. Laura Schlesinger.

26. Lund, S. & Renna, C. (2003), An analysis of the media response to the Spitzer study. *J. Gay & Lesbian Psychotherapy,* 7(3):55-67.

27. Editor's Note: See Spitzer, R. L. (2003), Reply: Study results should not be dismissed and justify further research on the efficacy of reparative therapy. *Archives Sexual Behavior,* 32(5):469-472. Reprinted in: *Ex-Gay Research: Analyzing the Spitzer Study and Its Relation to Science, Religion, Politics, and Culture,* ed. J. Drescher & K. J. Zucker. Binghamton, NY: The Haworth Press, 2006, pp. 223-231.

28. Stålström, O. & Nissinen, J. (2003), The Spitzer study and the Finnish parliament. *J. Gay & Lesbian Psychotherapy,* 7(3):83-95.

29. Wainberg, M.L, Bux, D., Carballo-Dieguez, A., Dowsett, G.W., Dugan, T., Forstein, M., Goodkin, K., Hunter, J., Irwin, T., Mattos, P., McKinnon, K., O'Leary, A., Parson, J. & Stein, E. (2003), Science and the Nuremberg Code: A question of ethics and harm. *Arch. Sexual Behavior,* 32(5):455-457.

SELECTED BIBLIOGRAPHY

Spitzer, R.L., Cohen, J., Fleiss, J.L. & Endicott, J. (1967), Quantification of agreement in psychiatric diagnosis: A new approach. *Arch. Gen. Psychiatry,* 17: 83-87.

Spitzer, R.L. & Fleiss, J.L. (1974), A re-analysis of the reliability of psychiatric diagnosis. *British J. Psychiatry,* 125:341-347.

Spitzer, R.L. (1976), More on pseudoscience in science and the case for psychiatric diagnosis: A critique of D.L. Rosenhan's "On Being Sane in Insane Places" and "The Contextural Nature of Psychiatric Diagnosis." *Arch. Gen. Psychiatry,* 33:459-470.

Spitzer, R.L., Endicott, J. & Robins, E. (1978), Research diagnostic criteria: Rationale and reliability. *Arch. Gen. Psychiatry,* 35:773-782.

Spitzer, R.L. & Williams, J.B.W. (1987), Introduction. In: *Diagnostic and Statistical Manual of Mental Disorders,* Third Edition, Revised (DSM-III-R). Washington, DC: American Psychiatric Association.

Spitzer, R.L., Gibbon, M., Skodol, A.E., Williams, J.B.W. & First, M.B. (1988), *DSM-III-R Case Book.* Washington, DC: American Psychiatric Press.

Spitzer, R.L. & Williams, J.B.W. (1988), Having a dream: A research strategy for DSM-IV. *Arch. Gen. Psychiatry,* 45:871-875. Reprinted in: *The Validity of Psychiatric Diagnosis,* ed. L. Robins. New York, Raven Press, 1989.

Spitzer, R.L., Williams, J.B.W., First, M.B. & Kendler, K.S. (1989), A proposal for DSM-IV: Solving the "organic/nonorganic problem." Editorial in *J. Neuropsychiatry,* 1(2):126-127.

Spitzer, R.L., Severino, S.K., Williams, J.B.W. & Parry, B.L. (1989), Late luteal phase dysphoric disorder and DSM-III-R. *American J. Psychiatry,* 146(7):892-897.

Spitzer, R.L., Williams, J.B.W., Gibbon, M. & First, M.B. (1992), The Structured Clinical Interview for DSM-III-R (SCID) 1: History, rationale and description. *Arch. Gen. Psychiatry,* 49:624-629.

Spitzer, R.L., Yanovski, S., Wadden, T., Wing, R., Marcus, M.D., Stunkard, A., Devlin, M.J., Mitchell, J., Hasin, D. & Horne, R. (1993), Binge eating disorder: Its further validation in a multisite study. *Intl. J. Eating Disorders,* 13:137-153.

Spitzer, R.L., First, M.B., Kendler, K.S. & Stein, D. (1993), The reliability of three definitions of bizarre delusions. *American J. Psychiatry,* 150:880-884.

Spitzer, R.L., Williams, J.B.W., Kroenke, K., Linzer, M., deGruy, F.V., Hahn, S.R., Brody, D. & Johnson, J.G. (1994), Utility of a new procedure for diagnosing mental disorders in primary care: The PRIME-MD 1000 Study. *JAMA,* 272: 1749-1756.

Spitzer, R.L., Kroenke, K., Williams, J.B.W. & the Patient Health Questionnaire Primary Care Study Group (1999), Validation and utility of a self-report version of PRIME-MD: The PHQ Primary Care Study. *JAMA,* 282:1737-1744.

Spitzer, R.L. (2001), Values and assumptions in the development of DSM-III and DSM-III-R: An insider's perspective and a belated response to Sadler, Hulgus, and Agich's "On Values in Recent American Psychiatric Classification." *J. Nerv. & Ment. Disease,* 189:351-359.

SECTION II:
THE EARLY FOUNDERS OF AGLP

Chapter 7

An Interview with Frank Rundle, MD

Richard O. Hire

JGLP: The *Journal of Gay & Lesbian Psychotherapy* is publishing a series of biographical interviews of pioneers in psychiatry who have made important contributions to gay and lesbian patients and their therapists. Because you are one of those pioneers, in fact a founding member of the Association of Gay and Lesbian Psychiatrists (AGLP), I've invited you here today. To start, could you tell me how you became interested in psychiatry?

DR. RUNDLE: Well, I grew up in a very small town of about 5,000 people in Montana, a real cow town, called Miles City. I'm the middle of five sons, and some time around the age of six I decided I would be a doctor; and I always thought that. When I was fourteen, we moved to Seattle, the first year of World War II, because there was work there for my father and older brother. I had the good fortune to end up in a very affluent suburb which had a very good school system, so I had a really extraordinary high school experience. I then went for four years to the University of Washington as a premed student. Those were the days when there were twenty applicants for every position, so the competition was really cutthroat. The first war veterans were coming back, they knew what they wanted, and they were really hard workers. First, I was accepted at the University of Washington, which had just opened its medical school, but then I was accepted by Northwestern. The University

This chapter appeared originally under the same title in *Journal of Gay & Lesbian Psychotherapy* 5(2):83-97. Copyright 2001 The Haworth Press, Inc.

American Psychiatry and Homosexuality: An Oral History
Published by The Haworth Press, Inc., 2007. All rights reserved.
doi:10.1300/6049_08

of Washington let me go and I studied for four years in Chicago. I worked while I was in school, in various places like the House of Corrections, and a hospital which was an all-male hospital. I worked as an extern in Evanston Hospital for a year, and graduated in 1953. I went into the Navy because the doctor draft law was still being enforced, and I did my internship in San Diego Naval Hospital, which was a really good experience. There, one of my electives was in psychiatry. All the psychiatrists were reservists who had trained at Menninger's, so I had a really great learning experience there. The chief of psychiatry that year was transferring to be chief at Bethesda, and he asked if I wanted to go. So I did.

I got married while I was in residency. At that time, of course, I believed that I was "sick" because of my homosexual feelings. And I thought if I got married that would all go away *[chuckle]*. I got married and soon afterward was transferred to Japan. There, really as less than a "half-baked" psychiatrist, I was put in charge of a thiry-bed acute treatment unit and a sixty-bed convalescent unit in a naval hospital.

JGLP: So, you were responsible for the care of ninety patients?

DR. RUNDLE: Yes, but I lucked out because the captain who was chief of service was an analyst who had been analyzed by Frieda Fromm-Reichman. He was a very smart guy and very permissive in letting me do things. Another staff person was a child psychiatrist trained at Payne Whitney, and there was a third guy who had trained at Montefiore. So I had a lot of supervision and a lot of teaching. Again, it was a great year, except for the fact that shortly after I got there, the infamous Office of Naval Intelligence conducted one of their sweeps, which they called "Operation Fishnet," looking for homosexuals. They hauled in—I don't know how many—dozens, scores of men. Many of them were corpsmen who worked on my unit, or yeomen who worked in the hospital. So I arrived at work one morning and found some of them on the unit as patients, and others in the brig. I had a real panic reaction, and depression. I got through that with the help of the Payne Whitney–trained psychiatrist. But it just opened my eyes to the vicious persecution to which gays in the military were subjected, like hiding tape recorders under the tatami mats in their Japanese houses, where many of them were living with Japanese women. There were some officers caught also. They all ended up either accepting discharge under less than honorable conditions or they were court-martialed.

JGLP: And this was solely for being caught in homosexual activity?

DR. RUNDLE: Yes, for being gay. So I finished the two years in Japan and went to Payne Whitney to finish my residency, primarily on the strength of the recommendation of the psychiatrist who was stationed there. At that time, Oscar Diethelm was chairman and he was a protégé of Adolph Meyer. He wasn't strictly a psychobiologist, but more of a psychopathologist. It was a good training program. My first year I was assigned seven patients, and I spent an hour a day with every one of them, even the mute catatonics and the psychotically depressed, who couldn't talk much either. I myself developed an episode of clinical depression and the professor sent me off to one of the analysts, which was not much help, but I got over it. I finished the residency in 1961 and went into private practice in Manhattan and stayed there for about a year. And I guess by that time, we had two children and were facing the issue of private school in Manhattan, a move to the suburbs, or a move elsewhere. We decided to move to Madison, Wisconsin, because we thought it would be a good place to raise children and it had good schools.

There I worked initially at the state hospital, which was an eye-opener because all of my training had been at Payne Whitney, which was a very isolated place—we got patients like Time-Life executives, senators and congresspeople, movie stars, and the rich people from Cuba and Venezuela. So my experience was limited. In the state hospital, I loved working with that population. I left after two years and then I worked half-time at a community mental health center and put together a group practice. We had about eighteen general psychiatrists, child psychiatrists, clinical psychologists, and social workers. Madison was a great town professionally. The level of care was just tops. We had a 300-bed hospital with over 400 board-certified specialists. That went on for four years, and then I fell in love with a young man, twenty years younger than me. I just knew that it was right, so I separated from my wife.

He and I moved to Monterey, California, and I took a job at Soledad Prison, which was very much in the news because of the Soledad brothers, whom you may remember: George Jackson and the others. Anyway, Jackson eventually admitted they killed the guard and dumped him off the third-floor tier. It was a very crazy place. Nobody trusted anybody. There were, I think, eighteen killings in a period of about eleven months. The guard was the first, then another guard, a number of inmates, and then while I was there, an inmate who was scheduled to meet with me killed one of their administrators in his office at the time he was supposed to be seeing me. So, this very paranoid administration believed that I was involved in this, that I had put him up to it, that I had supplied the weapon. They demanded that I give them his medical record, which I refused to do. So they fired me, and took his record plus some papers out of my briefcase that had nothing to do with him. Then I went into private practice in Monterey for about a year, and then to New York City to take a job with the prison health services of the City of New York's Department of Corrections. I was head of their department of psychiatry for about two years. Then I went to the Lower East Side Service Center, which is a drug treatment organization, and was there until 1977.

JGLP: When you worked at Soledad Prison was that your first prison work?

DR. RUNDLE: Yes.

JGLP: How did you decide to take that job?

DR. RUNDLE: Because it was near Monterey, thirty miles, and I thought I could work there full-time and start a part-time private practice and eventually do that full-time. But I got so caught up in the horrors that went on there.

I was assigned initially to what they called their "adjustment center," which is like super maximum security within the maximum-security section. People were locked up there for twenty-four hours a day for years, and some had been in solitary for ten years, and they were destroyed psychologically. Some were really brutalized physically, like keeping them naked in a concrete cell with water on the floor with no blanket and no mattress. It was just awful. And then a number of them who were in this unit had been there when the incident occurred which set off that whole Soledad brothers thing, which was the forced integration of these two maximum-security cell blocks—blacks, Mexicans, and whites. The very first time they put them out there in the exercise yard, three blacks and a white guy got into a fight and the guard shot three black prisoners dead and wounded the white guy. Three days later, a jury in Salinas ruled that this was justifiable homicide, and that's when the first guard got killed. Anyway, a bunch of these guys had been there, and I listened to their stories. All of their records had photographs of the dead ones—anyone who had been there at the time had photographs in their files—I saw them time and time again. One was shot through the heart. One, I think, the femoral artery was just torn out.

JGLP: These were photographs of the prisoners who had been killed in their files?

DR. RUNDLE: Yes, photographs of the dead inmates. I don't know why they put them in the inmates' records, but they did, and these guys talked to me about it. It was just mind-boggling. And then that the jury would say this was justifiable. The prisoners were in a fistfight! There were no weapons. And three black guys died and the white one lived.

JGLP: I sense that left a lasting impression on you.

DR. RUNDLE: It still upsets me. Jackson and the other two killed a guard, and a few months later, another guard was killed. In the meantime, inmates were killing each other, Mexicans killing blacks and blacks killing Mexicans, and the Aryan brotherhood killing both of them.

Then, before the administrator was killed that I told you about earlier, another guard from the maximum-security unit was stabbed in the neck with a pencil. He survived and they took him to the hospital, and, in my opinion, because of bad medical care he died. The wound bled through the tissues and cut off the carotid artery. And the guy who stabbed him was the inmate for whom I had been subpoenaed to testify about the conditions under which he was kept. He was the one kept naked in the flooded cell with no blanket and no mattress. And I just answered the questions which were put to me. The next day, when I went to work, I was met by an irate deputy superintendent who said the superintendent wanted to see me right away. He wanted to know why I had said those things. I said, I just answered the questions. Well, they wanted to fire me. But they didn't.

Then another incident happened. I became acquainted with a lawyer who formed a group that was trying to help prisoners. She arranged for a group called "The Committee for Public Justice" to visit the prison. This committee had been founded by Lillian Hellman after the Communist-baiting days in Hollywood. So, Lillian Hellman came with the psychiatrist Robert Coles, Roger Wilkins from the NAACP [National Association for the Advancement of Colored People], and Jane Moore, the wife of the Episcopal Bishop of New York. And I took them on a tour of the maximum-security section against the superintendent's wishes. Lillian Hellman, in her floor-length mink, in this maximum-security place which stank and was noisy, was hanging on my arm, saying, "Oh my God, I'm going to be sick. Get me out of here." But I got the administration further enraged that I would show these people that part of the prison. Then it was shortly after that the administrator was killed and they fired me.

JGLP: Because you wouldn't turn over the medical record?

DR. RUNDLE: Yes. Actually I pursued administrative remedy but got nowhere. I went to court and the judge ruled that the physical record belonged to the superintendent. That's now changed, but this was in 1972. Today, records belong to the medical department and are confidential, except in instances involving murder or escape. But the medical department is usually run by a retired military person who sees his loyalty to the superintendent, not to the patient.

JGLP: You mentioned earlier that you have children.

DR. RUNDLE: Yes. Three sons. When I divorced my wife, she was very angry and she told the kids I never sent them any money, which was a lie. I sent child support every month. So they grew up hating me. When they got into their teens, one by one they contacted me and wanted to meet and talk. They all pretty much said the same thing, that they knew I was gay. They had met my lover before I left Madison. I now feel accepted and okay with two of them. The eldest one is very straight-laced and married to a very church-religious kind of person. He has a hard time about it, I think, but he's not open about it. I see him and just spent a few days in Disney World with his family. I have six grandchildren, ages fifteen years old to seven.

JGLP: Have you enjoyed being a grandfather?

DR. RUNDLE: You know, initially I didn't like the idea, but, yes, I do. They're great kids and as a grandfather you are automatically a great person. I wish I could be around them more.

JGLP: Tell me about your initial involvement with AGLP?

DR. RUNDLE: In 1976, at the APA convention in Miami, I saw this scrawled sign for the GLB Caucus, and after a lot of pacing back and forth I went into this meeting. There were mostly residents or very young psychiatrists, except for Jim Paulsen. Jim and I became friends. At that same meeting, Barbara Giddings had an exhibit which she had been doing for several years. The theme of the exhibit was "long-term gay relationships." She used Damien Martin and Emery Hetrick as her subjects and had lots of photographs. So Jim and I would sit at that booth. A lot of people we both knew would come by, like former professors and teachers, and they would look aghast! Somehow I didn't feel anxious about that at all. It just seemed very matter-of-fact.

Just before that meeting, I had met Richard, who became my lover. And the other thing that happened in 1976 that probably changed the direction I went was volunteering at the St. Marks Health Clinic in New York, which treated a lot of gay men. We had a "gay night" on Monday, and we would see forty or fifty people. Those were the days when gonorrhea, syphilis, amebiasis, hepatitis B, and other STDs were rampant. But I got to know how badly gay men were treated by most doctors and most medical establishments.

Through Richard I got to know a group of people who went to Fire Island in the summer, so I became the doctor for the summer in the Pines between 1977 and 1979. Richard and I would have a house out there between May and September and I had an office in the city. Most of my patients were gay men. So for ten years, from 1977 to 1987, I did primary care, and not psychiatry, although there was obviously a lot of psychiatry involved. Richard died, probably a suicide, in 1981, of a cocaine overdose, which just about unhinged me. But I managed to keep working. In the meantime, we were developing AGLP. We went through several name changes.

Then, in 1977, the meeting was in Toronto and Jim and I both went, expecting we would have this organization meeting again. But there wasn't anything planned. Nobody had set it up. So Jim and I hastily put together a meeting. We didn't have very many attendees. And we just volunteered ourselves to be co-chairs of the caucus. So Jim was in San Francisco, I was in New York, and between 1977 and 1978, pretty much, it was I who organized the meeting at the APA in Atlanta in 1978. I planned the program and we were listed in the APA program schedule for the first time. Previously, meetings usually had been in gay bars.

So we had this organizing meeting in Atlanta at which about 100 people showed up. I had put ads in *Psychiatric News* and there were a lot of people who came who hadn't come to an APA meeting in years, gay men, and who were very interested in what was happening. It was a very chaotic, raucous meeting. First of all, someone wanted to know if anyone was there who wasn't gay, and some woman got up and announced she was there because she wanted to help us; she was from some evangelical Christian group. So they insisted that she leave. Then there were a lot of undercurrents, people who, I guess, really wanted to take over. Anyway, Jim and I survived that, and we and Richard Pillard and Emery Hetrick were elected officers of what was still called the Caucus of Gay, Lesbian, and Bisexual Psychiatrists of the APA. Then I think it got changed to the GLB Caucus of the APA. And then, at the APA meeting in Chicago in 1979, we had our first booth, our first exhibit. And we almost didn't have it because, I personally believe, the APA didn't want us to have it.

JGLP: What happened?

DR. RUNDLE: Kathleen O'Brian was the meetings management person. I had called her about setting up the exhibition booth and she said she would call me back. Then she left for Europe and didn't call me back. I called the program chairman. He said there was a big discussion going on that we shouldn't have "political exhibits" in our scientific program, but he said "I'll do what I can."

JGLP: This was six years after the diagnosis of homosexuality had been removed from the *Diagnostic and Statistical Manual* (DSM)?

DR. RUNDLE: Yes, in 1979 in Chicago. I forget the program chairman's name, but he was decent and he called back and said they had separated the political booths from the scientific booths. So our booth and the women's booth, and the Amnesty International were tucked away into a corner under the stairway. Our exhibit that year was called "The Visible, Invisible Psychiatrist." I had this gadget constructed which would flash, first, "Visible," then "Invisible." It was quite eye-catching.

We had a lot of opposition. We had it the previous year in Atlanta too. For example, the posters we put up in the hotel, in the convention, at the meeting sites, signs at our hotel suite, would be pulled off the wall. In Chicago, someone started what they called SCAPA, the Straight Caucus of the APA, and they left a bunch of their cards on our exhibit table. And we also had a nasty note left there that said things like, "We know you fag ass queers like flowers," something like that. I still have the note. But we had a really successful meeting at the caucus. People came, we had groups and meetings with a lot of participation.

Then, between 1979 and 1980, I worked on bylaws, because we didn't have any. We had no organization, we had no dues, we were surviving on contributions. The bylaws were accepted at the APA meeting in San Francisco in 1980, when David Kessler became president.

JGLP: You were president in 1978?

DR. RUNDLE: Well, from 1977 until 1980. We called the position "chairman" then. A very important thing happened politically in Atlanta in 1978. Jim and I met with Judd Marmor and with John Spiegel. John had been president of the APA, and in fact he came to our meeting in Atlanta to encourage us to organize, and he advised us to go to the Council on National Affairs and ask for a task force on gay and lesbian issues to be appointed. Judd Marmor advised us not to do that, but at the time John was chairman of the council. So I went to the council and made a statement that we had organized, and that we were requesting that a task force be appointed to look at gay, lesbian, and bisexual issues. After I made this very short statement, there was this loud whisper, "It's about time!" from a black female psychiatrist. So they were very supportive and were glad we were doing it.

Eventually the task force became the Committee on Gay, Lesbian, and Bisexual Issues. Jim Paulsen was the first chair. I was appointed, so was Richard Green, and I've forgotten the names of a couple of other people who were also appointed. Jim and I did most of the work. I served for five years, but after Richard (my lover) died in 1981, I just pretty much dropped out. Dave Kessler and Jim Krajeski and all the people who followed carried it on. Jim Krajeski was very important in his role as the APA assembly representative. He could be persuasive, rational, and not angry. I couldn't do that, without being confrontational and arousing opposition, so it was a good thing he was in there. And Dave Kessler was very important as well during that time. So that's how we got started.

JGLP: When did AGLP officially start?

DR. RUNDLE: Well, first of all, there was the whole issue of the caucus of the APA. In Chicago, in 1979, the APA sent some really repulsive public affairs guy to come to persuade us to change our name to Caucus of Members of the APA. They had already done it on their own, "they" being whoever ran and wrote about us in *Psychiatric News*. We were already being called "Caucus of Members of the APA" in *Psychiatric News,* but not with our permission. They didn't even talk to us. I didn't want to change the name, but the membership voted to go along with it, so we became the Caucus of Homosexually Identified Psychiatrists (CHIP). I don't know exactly when we became AGLP. It was after 1980. I think Jeanne Spurlock was instrumental in helping us to become established as a minority group, but I'm not sure exactly when that happened.

JGLP: Was she the individual who did the stage whisper at the Council on National Affairs?

DR. RUNDLE: No. Her name was ——. I'm sure she's known to many, a very outgoing, very strong woman who I think became an academic psychiatrist somewhere. In the early days, we had no organization, no dues, and we depended on contributions from individuals. Jim and I would rent the hospitality suites, which we would pay for because we would sleep there, and that went on for several years because we just didn't have the money. To get the reception, luncheons, and dinners set up with hotels, I would front the money, and eventually I would get it back, but it often took months. And then we had a crisis when the woman who was our treasurer didn't deposit checks for about eight months and suddenly I was getting all these inquiries from people asking why their checks hadn't cleared. It turns out she just hadn't deposited them. I pursued her and tried to get her to deposit them but she didn't do it. I finally went to Boston and threatened her that if she didn't deposit the checks I would get somebody after her. So she finally deposited them, but she's never forgiven me for that.

So we had lots of growing pains. I remember in Atlanta in 1978, my lover Richard was standing at the bottom of an escalator handing out flyers about our group and people coming down the escalator were kind of a captive audience. So they'd take them, and it was fun to watch. Some of them would give it back quickly; some would stop to read it after they got off. A lot of the hotel staff, like the room service people and the bus boys, would bring us food and things that were left over from other APA parties. And the printer I went to in Atlanta—a lot of gay people were working there and were cheering us on, would read the stuff that I'd bring in at night to have reproduced for the next day. It was very exciting. We truly are everywhere!

JGLP: When the AIDS crisis started, did that affect the organization?

DR. RUNDLE: Yes, it certainly did. We used to have a memorial service every year for all the people who died the previous year. In the years between 1981 and I guess around 1987, a lot of people died. I guess we don't have those services anymore. John Fryer used to be sort of the chaplain and Richard Nix played the organ or the piano. It had a big effect on me personally because so many of the people in my practice were young gay men and they were just dying.

JGLP: You were still working in New York at that time in primary care?

DR. RUNDLE: Yes. There was no treatment. There was no test for HIV. We didn't really know how it was transmitted in the early years. I just couldn't deal with all the deaths. When medical treatment for AIDS became available, I couldn't deal with the complexities of it. So that's when I decided to go back to psychiatry full-time, locum tenens. I've been doing that since 1986.

JGLP: Where are some of the places you've worked in locum tenens?

DR. RUNDLE: First I worked in Billings, Montana, at an adolescent treatment center and I've worked many times in the State Hospital in Warm Springs, Montana. Several times in the Wyoming State Hospital in Evanston. I've been to six of the seven regional treatment centers in Minnesota; Bakersfield, California; Logansport, Indiana; Hazard, Kentucky. Saratoga Springs—that was the best! I've worked in Nevada, both Reno and Las Vegas. I figure I've worked in about a hundred different places in the past fourteen years.

JGLP: Has being a psychiatrist who is gay ever come up as an issue in your work?

DR. RUNDLE: The people I work for in the locum tenens company know. I'm not sure how they know, except it just came up in conversation and I didn't try to hide it. But I haven't really encountered any negative situations. In fact, in the Montana adolescent treatment center, there was a fifteen-year-old kid who was obviously gay, who was being ridiculed and harassed and treated very badly, not only by the other kids, but by the staff. Without making it overt that I was gay, I think I was able to help him and support him and maybe give him some direction. But my being gay never became an issue. I don't volunteer, but if someone asked me I would certainly tell them. But it hasn't come up.

JGLP: It sounds like in your life as a psychiatrist, there have been two times when you've faced direct threats: in the armed services where you saw discrimination against service members, and the other place being in the APA.

DR. RUNDLE: Yes. When Richard Pillard gave up doing the caucus newsletter, which I think was in 1979 or 1980, Larry Mass volunteered to be the editor and my lover Richard was the graphics person. So the two of them would be in our apartment working on this newsletter. At the top of it, we put the statement of the APA to the effect that homosexuality per se is not a psychiatric disorder, and noted in several issues that that was as far as the APA went. And I think there was a lot of opposition in the APA Board of Trustees. I tried to register Richard as my spouse for the 1979 Chicago meeting, and I got back a very formal letter explaining that he was not my spouse so of course he couldn't register. But Herb Gant, who was the editor of *Psychiatric News,* told me they had a huge discussion about that in the board of trustees meeting, and everyone acknowledged that they were going to have to change that. So the APA changed it to "guests." Of course, in those days, there were many psychiatrists registering their female friends who were not their spouses.

JGLP: It's interesting that this past year the APA Auxiliary contacted the significant others group of AGLP to get more involved in the auxiliary. That's quite a change in twenty years!

DR. RUNDLE: Well, I'm sure there were many who would have supported us if they hadn't been closeted, and some who were closeted supported us with contributions. I encountered several who made that clear, saying, "I can't support you the way I'd like to, but here's a check," which was fine because we needed that support too. Of course many of the gay staff who worked at the APA came to our parties and were supportive. It was like a safe place for them.

JGLP: It sounds as though things today are very different than they were twenty years ago. Do you have any thoughts about the direction AGLP is going?

DR. RUNDLE: I do wonder in what direction this organization will go. I think it is very important to do whatever we can do to encourage the medical students and residents to become involved, to know that we exist and that there are other people. I think there's a lot to be done yet about curriculum, especially in residency training and medical school. When I was in New York, the OB/GYN doctor who ran the human sexuality course invited me every year to appear before the freshman class at Mount Sinai. And that was really a wonderful experience each time, although not always pleasant because some of the students were pretty hostile.

JGLP: What would you talk about?

DR. RUNDLE: Well, I would talk about myself and how I happen to be where I am. About getting married and having kids, and then coming to acknowledge and understand that I was gay, which really changed my life tremendously. And the students were generally very curious and interested, usually empathetically, though some of them with hostility, but mostly not. I really enjoyed doing that, and I think we should do more of it. And then there is the whole issue of discrimination in academic institutions. I don't know how the organization can approach that, but it's surely there. The people who don't get promoted, who get fired, or don't get tenure. Jim Paulsen, for years, was working on a project to find people who thought they had been harmed by therapy with psychiatrists (doing reparative therapy). I don't know what happened to the material he collected. He had a homophobic son, and when he died, the son destroyed a lot of his stuff, and I got just a very small portion of it that his daughter salvaged.

JGLP: As you look back on your career from this point, what would you consider your most valuable contribution has been?

DR. RUNDLE: Well, actually I think it's been my involvement as an expert in litigation against prisons and jails and a few mental hospitals. I've been an expert in nearly 200 cases, about eighty-five of which were tried in Federal District Court, against single prisons,

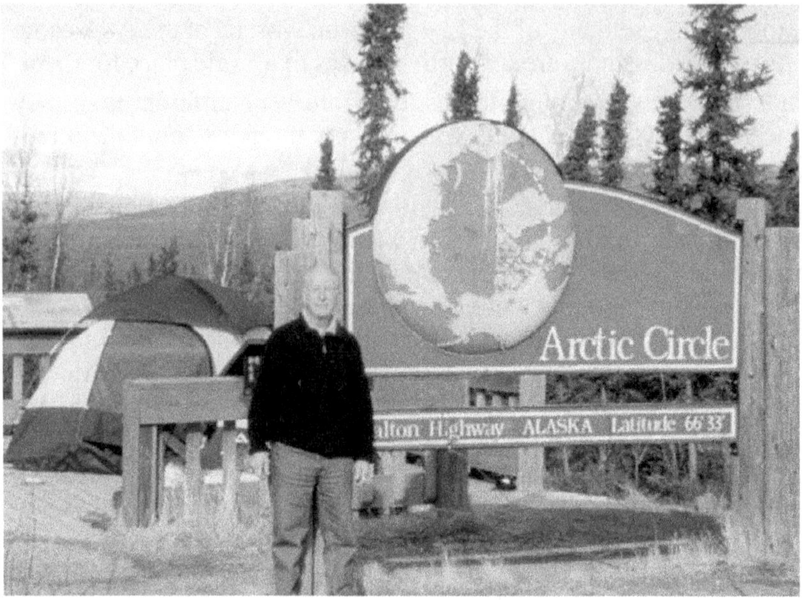

and state systems, like Texas, Alabama, Oklahoma. I think real significant changes came out of that work.

JGLP: Were these cases about health issues?

DR. RUNDLE: Initially they were about general conditions, like overcrowding and lack of exercise, guard brutality, lack of training or educational opportunities, and bad medical care or no medical care. These were mostly in the 1970s, and we won them all. The Department of Justice used to have a special litigation section, in the Civil Rights Division, which was actively suing states and prisons and mental hospitals, and they won those cases. And the national prison project of the ACLU [American Civil Liberties Union] also brought a lot of those cases and they won most of them. When the general conditions issues became less of a concern, then medical care, mental health care, and suicide in institutions became a focus. And until Reagan became president and disbanded that special litigation section, there were a lot of suits brought and a lot of change occurred.

Now it's almost impossible. Congress passed what they call "Prison Reform Litigation," something which makes it almost im-

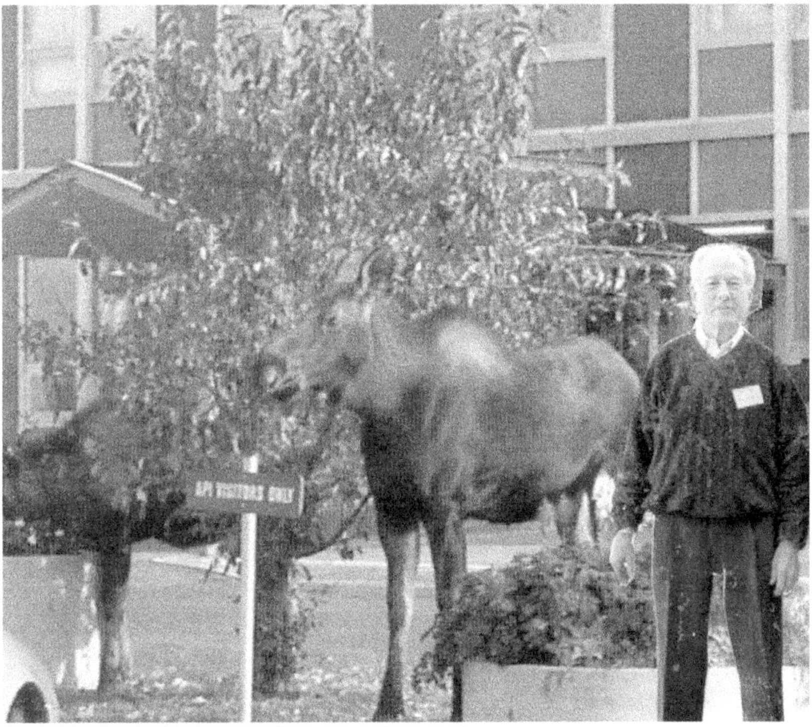

possible to sue them, for any reasons. The last suit I was involved with was a few years ago, when Alabama brought the chain gang back. The Southern Poverty Law Center sued them and got together experts like Norman Carlson, who was the director of the Federal Bureau of Prisons for thirty years, who became an expert in testifying against these chain gangs. And a professor of law from the University of Chicago, myself, and a lot of correctional people were involved. And they won that case. Other than that, I haven't had a request to get involved for years.

I think that just in terms of the numbers of people whose lives were made easier, I think that work was the most important thing, but if I think about gay people, I think that my work with this organization [AGLP] is the most important.

JGLP: It seems there are more and more people in jail now with psychiatric and substance abuse disorders.

DR. RUNDLE: Yes, there's no question about it. There are a few states which have taken new initiatives to develop treatment centers, or have been forced to by courts. New York is one. Another lawsuit I was involved with involved what they called "The Hospital for the Criminally Insane," which was run by the Department of Corrections up in Beacon, New York. The court ordered that closed. A new place was opened in Marcy, which was actually quite a good psychiatric treatment center. But it's just not big enough. I'm still going to New York as a monitor for a federal judge in a case involving a women's prison in Bedford Hills. I've been going now for twenty years, trying to get them to conform to the judge's orders. I used to go four times a year, but now I'm down to two or three times a year. I'll be going in July. I think that will be my next to last visit because they finally got medical care up to an acceptable standard. They fought, dragged their feet, which is typical of prison litigation. Twenty years is not unusual.

JGLP: I really appreciate your sharing so much of your life today. I've found much of what you've shared fascinating and inspiring.

DR. RUNDLE: There's so much to try to say and so much doesn't get said.

Chapter 8

An Interview with David R. Kessler, MD

Mary E. Barber

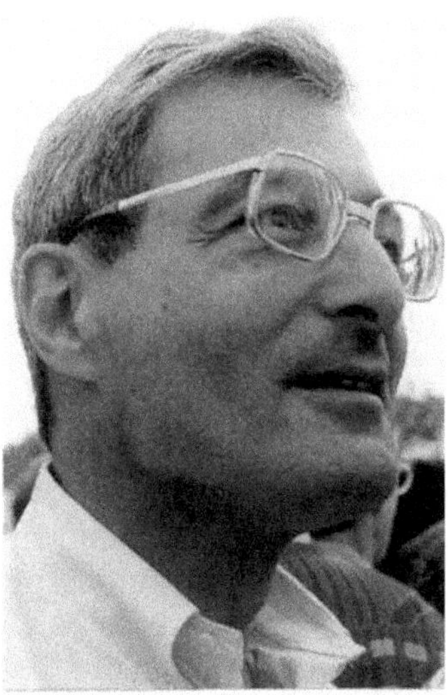

David R. Kessler, MD, was the first elected president of the San Francisco–based gay doctors group—Bay Area Physicians for Human Rights (BAPHR)—from 1978 to 1980. He was reelected BAPHR's president in 1988. From 1980 to 1982, he was president of what is today known as the Association of Gay and Lesbian Psychiatrists (AGLP), in the days when the group functioned as a gay caucus within the American Psychiatric Association. He has been a member of the boards of directors of the National Gay and Lesbian Task Force and the NAMES Project.

Dr. Kessler endowed the David R. Kessler Lectures in Lesbian and Gay Studies at the Center for Lesbian and Gay Studies (CLAGS) of the City University of New York (CUNY). This series, the first of its kind at an academic institution, has honored prominent figures in the lesbian and gay community with an annual lecture since its inception in 1992. Past honorees have included Edmund White, Judith Butler, Samuel Delany, Eve Kosofsky Sedgwick, and John D'Emilio. The first ten Kessler lectures have been published as a book (CLAGS, 2003).

American Psychiatry and Homosexuality: An Oral History

doi:10.1300/6049_09

Dr. Kessler completed his medical degree at Yale in 1955, and his psychiatry residency at Yale in 1961. He was on the faculty of the Department of Psychiatry at the University of California San Francisco Medical School and on the full-time staff of the Langley Porter Institute from 1962 until his retirement as Clinical Professor of Psychiatry in 1986. His other professional role has been as a forensic psychiatrist consulting to the California courts, work which has continued after his retirement. *JGLP* spoke with Dr. Kessler by phone from his San Francisco home.

JGLP: Tell us about your background.

DR. KESSLER: I am an only child of an eldest son; that probably tells you something about me right there. I was raised in Brooklyn, where I went to high school and then to Brooklyn College, and enjoyed New York's cultural activities. I recommend people live in New York, at least for a while. The first time I was away from home for an extended period, except for summer camp, was when I went off to Yale Medical School in 1951. That had a profound effect on my life. I began to see what the rest of the world was like. I cannot say I thoroughly enjoyed all of medical school, but I certainly liked the atmosphere and the surroundings.

I've been lucky in the friends I've made over the years. For example, I met Marty Duberman while I was at Yale later for my psychiatric residency. As you know, he is now a well-known professor, author and playwright, and the founder of the Center for Lesbian and Gay Studies (CLAGS) at the City University of New York. At that time, he was an instructor in the Department of History at Yale, and there was a small closeted group of gay faculty to whom I was introduced. It was an interesting experience—all of us deeply closeted.

JGLP: How did you find each other?

DR. KESSLER: I think it was through a mutual friend, a psychologist in New York, who told me about Marty. I have known Marty for over forty years now. Another fortunate friendship was with one of my medical school classmates, Alan Stone, who later became president of the American Psychiatric Association (APA) in the same year that I was president of the GLB Caucus. And my closest friend back in junior high school and high school days was Ted Nadelson, who recently passed away. He became a psychiatrist and his wife, Carol Nadelson, became the first woman president of the APA. Also about forty years ago, I met Larry Kramer, who at that time was a Hollywood screenwriter (*Women in Love,* etc.), but has since gone on to great notoriety for his writing and AIDS activism. So I have been fortunate in knowing people who have been very helpful to me in my gay-related activities.

Anyway, back to Yale. I had gone to medical school to become a psychiatrist. But before that was possible, I had to get through all those other medical school subjects—you remember what that was like! After graduation, I faced the prospect of a a compulsory military service obligation, and so I interned with the U.S. Public Health Service in New York City. That is when I first came out in the gay world. As part of my rotating internship, I was on pediatrics at Lenox Hill Hospital in New York. One day, I was singing some arias from *Don Giovanni* in the shower. One of the other interns heard me and decided I must be gay. He was right, of course! He did not waste much time, and that's when I came out in the gay world and learned what the gay scene in New York was like. I did not come out publicly until quite a bit later.

I finished my internship and then spent two more years with the Public Health Service. One of those years was in the San Francisco Bay Area, which I found very appealing. Five years later, I came back. First I went back to Yale for my psychiatric residency. I was still in the closet but enjoyed my psychiatric training very much. I worked under a mentor who understood that I was gay and was quite supportive. He was from Hungary and gloried in the role of the continental sophisticate. I think he enjoyed the idea that he knew I was gay and that we had our little secret. So, that was basically a positive environment.

After residency, I stayed on the faculty as chief resident and instructor in psychiatry for a year but decided that I did not want to get too comfortable in New Haven. I had a boyfriend who lived in Philadelphia and worked for Dupont in Delaware. He was not too happy with his job, and I did not want to remain in New Haven forever. We put our heads together and thought, "Were shall we go? San Francisco, of course!" So we packed up and moved to San Francisco in 1962.

JGLP: Was San Francisco the gay mecca then that it is now?

DR. KESSLER: Yes. Bars and bathhouses were being raided from time to time, but there was quite a nucleus of gay people and there were some beginning gay and lesbian organizations. Things were percolating. By no means was life perfectly comfortable in San Francisco, but by comparison to other places, it was paradise.

I've been in San Francisco ever since 1962. I was able to walk into a staff position at the UC Psychiatry Department here, just the kind of job I was suited for, on a psychiatric inpatient service at the Langley Porter Institute. I stayed on the faculty full-time until I retired in 1986. The other part of my professional life has been forensic consultation to the criminal courts, which still continues on a part-time basis.

JGLP: What kinds of consultation do you do?

DR. KESSLER: Evaluations for mental competency to stand trial, or, occasionally, evaluations with regard to issues of legal sanity. I like forensic work because it is suitable for working part-time, and I can live vicariously through the stories I hear. Also, when I testify in court, I can release some of my exhibitionistic proclivities!

JGLP: Is it true you were involved in the Patty Hearst case?

DR. KESSLER: I was scheduled to be one of the prosecution's psychiatrist experts in the case. It was agreed that there would be three experts for the defense and three for the prosecution. I was to be the last examiner to interview Patty. By the time all the others were done with their lengthy examinations, Ms. Hearst, according to her attorneys' declarations to the court, was complaining of excessive harassment and stress. The federal judge then ruled that no more interviews would be permitted. So I became a psychiatric consultant to the U.S. Attorney's Office on the case. I worked with the prosecution, sat in on all the psychiatric testimony, but never testified.

JGLP: Did being gay ever come up as an issue in your work?

DR. KESSLER: Only a few times that I can think of in my career. One time in a federal case, I had evaluated a woman defendant, and the defense lawyer challenged me in court, saying something like, "How can Dr. Kessler know anything about women—because he's gay?"

JGLP: Did that have anything to do with the case?

DR. KESSLER: No, homosexuality had no relevance to the case, but he was trying to make a point that I could not be knowledgeable about the defendant because she was a woman. The judge knew me, as it happened. I had worked with him on the Patty Hearst case when he had been in the U.S. Attorney's Office. He said, "I know Dr. Kessler, and he is an experienced psychiatric expert, and your argument is irrelevant." It backfired on the lawyer because all this occurred in front of the jury! There were a couple of other times that people tried to make an issue of my being gay, but luckily each time someone was present who knew me and immediately defended me.

That's what I have been doing professionally over the years. I co-authored a textbook, *Marital and Family Therapy* (Glick and Kessler, 1974). My co-author was divorced and I was gay. What other people were better qualified to write a book on marital and family therapy?

JGLP: Of course! I am interested in your history with the Gay Caucus of the APA. Is that what it was called? I have heard different versions.

DR. KESSLER: The caucus had a lot of different names, which is an interesting story too. When the pioneers Frank Rundle,[1] Jim Paulsen, Richard Pillard,[2] and others got the group organized back in the 1970s, I think it was the GLB Caucus of the APA. My old friend, Mel Sabshin, past medical director of the APA, objected to that name. As I recall, the objection was that it sounded as though the organization was an official body of the APA, which it was not.

So we had to change the name to Gay Caucus of *Members* of the APA. It seems a little unimportant now in retrospect, but we went through a big hassle about that. Part of the problem was that at that point the APA was very sensitive about any implication that it was officially sponsoring a gay organization. I became aware of the Gay Caucus, I think, at the Atlanta annual meeting in 1978.

JGLP: The year that AGLP was formed.

DR. KESSLER: That's right. That was the year that we adopted bylaws and got officially organized. Before that it had been a loose, unofficial organization. There had been informal meetings of gay psychiatrists, often in gay bars or restaurants, at the time of the APA annual meetings. Frank Rundle and Jim Paulsen had been appointed co-chairs, because they were the most active—and probably because nobody else wanted to do all the work. It was not until 1978 that we adopted bylaws and had an election for president.

Just before that annual meeting, in that same year, Jim Paulsen and other "out" gay mental health professionals had come to the Langley Porter Institute to give a grand rounds on the topic of homosexuality. A lesbian social worker and I had gotten together to sponsor the grand rounds. With much trepidation and anxiety, we would meet, as secretly as possible, to plan the program. My heart was pounding during these meetings, afraid that somebody might see us and think that I was gay.

At about the same time, Anita Bryant was organizing a crusade from Florida to protect children from the evils of homosexuality. In California, a state senator sponsored a ballot initiative to ban openly gay teachers and any positive information about homosexuality in the public schools. The gay community responded with a massive political campaign. I remember being very angry and became involved in helping to organize a gay doctors group in San Francisco to fight the negative stereotyping of gay people. The group was named the Bay Area Physicians for Human Rights (BAPHR), and in 1978 I was elected president.

I began thinking to myself, "You know, it is going to be only a short time before you have to come out publicly. Why don't you use that grand rounds to come out to your department?" That may now sound more courageous (or outrageous!) than it actually was. After all, I was well established in my job, and I was in San Francisco. I did not have a private practice to worry about. I did not think anything terrible was going to happen to me, so I could take the chance and do it. I then decided that I would ask a question during the discussion period, but I would preface it with the phrase, "As a longtime gay psychiatrist myself . . ."

Which is exactly what I did. I do not remember what question I asked, but I do recall the preface. All the department faculty were there, the chairman was presiding, and it was also being televised and transmitted to other UC campuses. So I came out to all the UC psychiatry departments in California in one fell swoop.

JGLP: Do you remember that moment?

DR. KESSLER: I remember that moment very well. I was sweating with anxiety, but I was determined to do it. I knew it would be known sooner or later, now that I was head of the gay doctors' group. We would be marching in the Gay Pride Parade in a few months. The grand rounds seemed like a golden opportunity, so I grabbed it, although I did not know what kind of reception I'd get.

Interestingly, some of my colleagues never mentioned it. Never said a word. Others came over and said, "It's about time you did that. Good for you." My department chairman, who was an orthodox psychoanalyst, was not too pleased. Still, I suffered no lasting bad effects from that, I must say.

JGLP: It must have given you a lot of courage.

DR. KESSLER: Exactly, yes. It was a good first step, and, I figured, this has gone pretty well—I can just keep going. Soon after the grand rounds, the gay doctors participated in the 1978 San Francisco Gay Pride Parade. We marched with our banner, Bay Area Physicians for Human Rights. At that time, many gays, even in San Francisco, were still in the closet. The general public thought that only interior decorators, ballet dancers, and hairdressers were gay. Now here was a gay doctors' group marching in the parade, and we got lots of applause from the onlookers. It was really an important political statement as well as an ego booster, marching down Market Street, the main street in town, with people cheering and hollering. It was wonderful.

The next day, the *San Francisco Chronicle* ran a story saying something like, "Included in the parade yesterday were various groups *supportive* of gay rights, including doctors." The reporters apparently could not believe that there actually might be gay doctors. They characterized us as doctors who were in support of gay rights.

And this was not an uncommon experience. For example, one time Jim Krajeski[3] and I went to Las Vegas to attend an American Medical Association meeting about gay health issues. In passing, we mentioned the gay doctors' group in San Francisco. During the break, a friendly physician came over and said, "I'm a physician from Missouri, and I was interested in your presentation. You talked about a gay doctors' group in San Francisco. Well, that's very interesting. I know you guys have some gay doctors in San Francisco, but I can assure you that there are no gay doctors in Missouri." Hardly anyone knew any openly gay people in those years, as hard as it may be to believe now. It is hard to think back to that period in which gay people were basically invisible. So becoming increasingly visible became part of our strategy, one we borrowed from Harvey Milk.[4] His advice was to organize and come out, to do away with this invisibility of gay people.

Later, if you can believe it, there was a story about me in *People* magazine (Faber, 1979). It was my fifteen seconds of fame. It was not because it was me personally, but because I was part of a "gay doctors' group." I mean, who had ever heard of such a thing?

Incidentally, I had another few seconds of fame after Harvey Milk's death. I was asked to be one of the eulogists at his memorial service because someone considered a doctor to be respectable, I suppose. My friend Larry Kramer was in San Francisco at the time and made some suggestions about the draft of my speech. When he got back to New York he wrote an op-ed piece in the *New York Times* (Kramer, 1978) in his usual outspoken style, about how closeted and ineffective the gay community was in New York, and how he had just returned from San Francisco where they had a moving memorial for Harvey Milk, and he quoted from my remarks, which he had helped to write![5]

I was the first president of the Bay Area Physicians from 1978 to 1980. During that time, I started coming out all over the place at the annual APA meetings. For example, I remember that one of my former instructors ran into me at the meeting in 1979 and said, "Well, Dave, nice to see you. What're you doing?" I said, "Oh, I'm busy with the GLB Caucus." That took care of that! Some of us would sit at the GLB Caucus booth in the exhibit area, and colleagues would come by and do a double take when they saw our sign. So, it was easy to come out in wholesale fashion.

After two years of being president of the Bay Area Physicians, I became president of the GLB Caucus in 1980. By that time, we had a newsletter and an organizational structure. We were asking the APA for membership in the Council on National Affairs and for representation as a minority group in the APA Assembly. We got all that accomplished after a bit of a struggle, with lots of help from friends. Some of them I have already mentioned, but there are others: a semicloseted former president of the APA was very helpful; Judd Marmor[6] and John Spiegel, both former presidents of the APA, were remarkably supportive. It turned out later, by the way, that Spiegel himself was gay; he came out to his family many years later. There were many people—gay and straight, closeted and otherwise—who were helpful to us all along the way.

JGLP: Were you involved with, or aware of, the process that went on a few years earlier with the deletion of the diagnosis of homosexuality from the DSM?

DR. KESSLER: That was in 1973, and in those years, I was closeted. The word "gay" would send shivers up and down my spine. The removal of the diagnosis hardly registered on me somehow. It is remarkable because only a few years later I was out of the closet and activated. It was an amazing transformation, like personal nuclear fission. I do not know where all that energy came from, but, having been bottled up for so long, it had to emerge sooner or later.

[Even after the diagnosis' deletion] we had our struggles. In the early 1980s, when I was head of the GLB Caucus, we still had psychoanalysts telling us that although the APA may have deleted homosexuality per se from the manual, we were still sick, or at least had an arrested development. And many of the textbooks still had all kinds of horrible things to say about homosexuality.

JGLP: And there was still ego-dystonic homosexuality.[7]

DR. KESSLER: Right. So there was still plenty of work to do. We also had other goals in mind for our group. One was to act as a social support network for our own members. Another was to reduce the mystification about who gay people were. Just coming out and showing people who we were was eye-opening for our colleagues. Many of them, including important members of the DSM Nomenclature Committee, had never met, talked to, or taken a meal with an openly gay psychiatrist before. They were surprised to learn people they had known for years were actually gay and seemed pretty normal! I saw this as a very important part of what we were all about.

JGLP: What was the group like then? Was it mostly men?

DR. KESSLER: We always had problems with recruiting and retaining women, I think understandably. There were so many more men, and women felt outnumbered. We thought we were quite sensitive to the issue and leaning over backward to make women feel welcome, but perhaps we were not. Women felt they just did not have a real voice in the group, and so they would drop out. That was an ongoing challenge.

I am glad to see women in leadership positions now, and representing us in the assembly. It is a lot better than it used to be.

JGLP: I imagine there were psychiatrists in the group that were uncomfortable about the openness? Or that really were not able to be open?

DR. KESSLER: Yes, there always were, and I am sure there still are to this day. That was fine with me. We wanted to support them and make them feel that there was a place for them. If they felt uncomfortable about coming out in their communities or to other APA members, that was understandable. We wanted to be encouraging, but we felt we were not in a position to preach to them.

We would have, and you still have of course, the reception at the APA meetings in which the APA officers and lots of others come to politic. That is a mixed group—everybody can feel comfortable there—gay, closeted, straight, or whoever you are. Our goal was to make room for everybody and not think of our group as exclusively for openly gay people. There were plenty of opportunities for closeted gay psychiatrists and others to help us out. For instance, we had friends inside the APA, from whom we got useful advice and information. Such people could be of enormous help to us.

JGLP: And you could be of help to them.

DR. KESSLER: Exactly. The slogan used to be, "We are everywhere," and I remember one of our early meetings, I think it was in Chicago back in 1979. We were running short of money for the refreshments at our hospitality suite. We had had so many visitors to the hospitality suite for our social and educational functions that we were just overwhelmed. We were talking about this, I guess, and soon one of the gay hotel bellhops went around to other parties and scooped up the remains of their hors d'oeuvres and brought them to our suite. Also, we did some printing—posters, flyers, bulletins and the like. The printing company was gay-owned, and when they saw the content of what we were printing, they said, "Good, good, go, go!" So gay people really are everywhere!

I was president of the GLB Caucus for two years—1980 to 1982. The second year was kind of a fluke. If I remember correctly, in 1981 the APA was scheduled to meet in New Orleans. Well, Louisiana was one of the states opposed to the Equal Rights Amendment, which was a hot topic at that time. We had been petitioning the APA to boycott New Orleans because it was not in support of women's rights. The APA said that they had made commitments years in advance and could not change them at this late date. So the APA went on to New Orleans, and we joined with the American Academy of Psychoanalysis and a few other groups who decided to boycott New Orleans and hold their meetings in Houston. As it turned out, not all of our people went to Houston, and so there was some question about the succession of the caucus presidency. I just opted to stay on another year, sort of like a Latin American dictator.

By that time, our organization was pretty well connected to the APA and was solidly organized. We were gaining steadily in membership, and it seemed as if we were going to progress through our infancy and childhood in a healthy fashion. Still, I have been absolutely amazed to see just how well the group has advanced over the years. I have been delighted at the magnificent work it has been doing, thanks to people who have taken leadership roles and thanks to the support of the regular members.

JGLP: And of course we're all standing on the shoulders of everybody who started it all.

DR. KESSLER: Well, we all stand on the shoulders of others. That's the way it goes. Without Frank Rundle, Jim Paulsen, and Richard Pillard, we would not be talking today.

JGLP: Tell me about the CLAGS lecture series that you sponsor and how that came about.

DR. KESSLER: About fifteen years or so ago, I got to thinking that lots of wealthy gay people were dying of AIDS. I began to wonder what these people had done with the money they had left. I thought that money could be put to some good use for our community. Then I remembered that, at Yale, various wealthy people had endowed lectureships of one sort or another—the "So-and-So Lectures in the Arts," the "So-and-So Lectures in Science."

I put those two thoughts together, the money and the lectureships that I had attended and enjoyed, and decided to see if I could endow a lectureship at Yale. Why Yale? Well, I had connections to Yale. I also thought it would be very prestigious, in that the association of Yale and homosexuality would send a powerful positive public message.

JGLP: It would create such a high level of visibility.

DR. KESSLER: Just the way previously I thought that coming out as a gay doctor would give being gay a little bit of clout. So I thought similarly with this lectureship. When I went back to New Haven for a medical class reunion, I arranged to meet with the people in the Yale grants office about the possibility of funding such a program. However, it soon became clear to me that they were not quite ready for the idea. They listened politely, but they never got back to me with any proposals or tangible assistance. They indicated that there was no convenient administrative niche for such a program, and I also got the impression that there was no nucleus of openly gay faculty there who would support it.

I thought, "It's not going to work, not right now at Yale, so now what?" I then recalled that my old buddy Marty Duberman was by that time the founder and director of the Center for Lesbian and Gay Studies at the City University of New York. I also had another connection, in that CUNY also incorporates Brooklyn College, where I did my undergraduate work. New York City certainly seemed like a convenient location, where lots of people could attend such a lecture.

Well, CLAGS was very happy to hear that somebody wanted to give them money. At first, they did not know quite what to do administratively. I don't think anybody had offered to give them any money before. Eventually we got the paperwork straightened out, and the first lecture took place in 1992. A selection committee picks someone who has made an important contribution to the lives of gay and lesbian people. The talks draw an enthusiastic audience. I have been back to about half of these lectures over the years and it is just wonderful. I feel very fortunate to have been in a position to get that going, but I actually intended it as a demonstration project. I wanted other gay people to follow suit and contribute their money for other worthy projects—that was the whole idea. Where was all this gay money going? Well, I still do not know, but, anyway, Larry Kramer finally managed to persuade Yale to accept his idea for the Larry Kramer Initiative. That is funded, and up and running now. They sponsor various gay programs and I think they have a visiting professorship. Now there are other departments of gay and lesbian studies around the country, and that is good, but there is probably still a lot of gay money going down the drain that could be put to good use.

JGLP: It sounds like you started something.

DR. KESSLER: I was glad to be in a position to do something. When the discussions with Yale were going nowhere, I was afraid it would not happen, but then CLAGS picked up the ball and ran with it.

So you can see that one of the threads that runs through this whole story has to do with my good fortune in knowing all kinds of helpful people over the years.

JGLP: I am sure they've been lucky to know you as well.

DR. KESSLER: I don't know; you'd better ask them about that!

JGLP: And what else are you doing now? Are you enjoying your retirement?

DR. KESSLER: Well, I've gone back to playing the piano. I'm studying to be a prodigy! I do a little gardening, and I travel and see friends, and just enjoy life. I tell everybody I meet who is working that it's time for them to retire. They hate me!

JGLP: It's been a pleasure talking with you. Thanks for giving us a little window into your life and experiences.

DR. KESSLER: Thank you, too, because this has been an opportunity to go back into my memory and relive some of my past. I have not thought about much of this for quite a while, so it has been refreshing and enlivening for me to revisit these experiences.

NOTES

1. See Richard Hire's interview with Frank Rundle, MD, Chapter 7 in this book.

2. See Paul Lynch's interview with Richard C. Pillard, MD, Chapter 15 in this book.

3. James Krajeski, MD, is a longtime AGLP member and one of its past presidents. Dr. Krajeski is presently editor of the APA newspaper, *Psychiatric News.*

4. Harvey Milk was an openly gay city supervisor in 1970s San Francisco, shot to death by a political rival. His life story is told in Shilts, R. (1982), *The Mayor of Castro Street: The Life and Times of Harvey Milk.* New York: St. Martin's Press.

5. ". . . Dr. David Kessler, psychiatrist on the staff of the University of California Medical School and the Langley Porter Psychiatric Clinic, and president of the Bay Area Physicians for Human Rights, a group of more than 250 homosexual doctors and psychiatrists, spoke. 'Harvey asked us all to come out to our families and friends, to the people we work with and to those we shop from . . . so that we can shatter the myth, once and for all, that we were freaks, weirdos, or sickies. . . . Harvey Milk fought for us. Now it is our turn to fight for him.' Inside the Opera

House, 4,000 people rose as one to shout." The piece concludes with, "Harvey Milk . . . Dr. David Kessler—we have no one like you here" (Kramer, 1978).

6. See Vernon Rosario's interview with Judd Marmor, MD, Chapter 5 in this book.

7. Ego-dystonic homosexuality was in the DSM-III (APA, 1980) and removed from the DSM-III-R (APA, 1987) in 1987.

REFERENCES

American Psychiatric Association (1980), *Diagnostic and Statistical Manual of Mental Disorders,* Third Edition. Washington, DC: American Psychiatric Press.

American Psychiatric Association (1987), *Diagnostic and Statistical Manual of Mental Disorders,* Third Edition—Revised. Washington, DC: American Psychiatric Press.

CLAGS (2003), *Queer Ideas: The David R. Kessler Lectures in Lesbian and Gay Studies.* New York: Feminist Press.

Faber, N. (1979), Medics: Psychiatrist D. Kessler. *People Magazine,* 11(May 21): 101-102.

Glick, I.D. & Kessler, D.R. (1974), *Marital and Family Therapy.* New York: Grune & Stratton.

Kramer, L. (1978), Gay "power" here. *The New York Times,* December 13, p. 27.

Chapter 9

An Interview with Nanette Gartrell, MD

Mary E. Barber

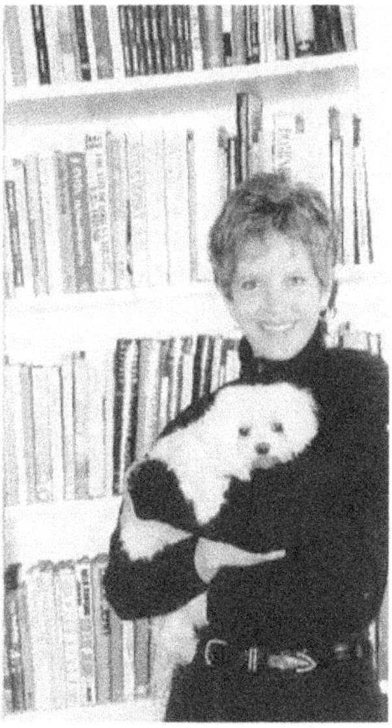

Nanette Gartrell, MD, is known for her research on sexual abuse of patients by psychiatrists, done in the 1980s, research that was instrumental in changing ethics codes for medicine and psychiatry. Her National Longitudinal Lesbian Family Study has been proceeding since 1986, giving a rich window into the lives of a group of lesbian mothers and their children. She maintains a private practice in San Francisco, where she also writes and conducts her research.

In the late 1970s and early 1980s, Dr. Gartrell was one of the pioneering members of the Association of Gay and Lesbian Psychiatrists (AGLP). Along with Peggy Hanley-Hackenbruk, MD, and others, Dr. Gartrell paved the way for more women to be involved in AGLP. Dr. Gartrell was a member of the American Psychiatric Association (APA) Committee on Women for several years during the 1980s and

Dr. Barber wishes to acknowledge the assistance of Elie Gruber in preparing this interview.

This chapter appeared originally under the same title in *Journal of Gay & Lesbian Psychotherapy* 7(4):35-47. Copyright 2003 The Haworth Press, Inc.

American Psychiatry and Homosexuality: An Oral History
Published by The Haworth Press, Inc., 2007. All rights reserved.
doi:10.1300/6049_10

served as committee chair from 1982 to 1984. She has also had many years of involvement with the lesbian physicians' group Women in Medicine.

Dr. Gartrell completed her undergraduate degree in biology at Stanford University in 1972, then went on to medical school at UC Davis. She did her psychiatric training at two Harvard-affiliated programs: her psychiatry residency at the Massachusetts Mental Heath Center and a consultation-liaison fellowship at Beth Israel Hospital. She then remained on the faculty at Harvard from 1979 to 1988 before moving to UC–San Francisco, where she has remained since 1988.

The *Journal of Gay & Lesbian Psychotherapy* interviewed Dr. Gartrell in the office of her lavender townhouse, located in the Laurel Heights neighborhood of San Francisco. Dr. Gartrell began by speaking about being the first "out" lesbian on the Harvard Medical School faculty, and of being a feminist in a generally male-dominated environment.

JGLP: Did you run into conflict being on the faculty and wanting to study things from that point of view?

DR. GARTRELL: Always! I've always found it interesting to recall that, in those years, I seemed to have a lot more frustration with responses to my feminism than responses to my lesbianism, and I think it's probably about the attitude I have in trying to educate people. Whenever people made homophobic comments, I automatically went into educational mode. I would just power down, become very thoughtful, and then pull out as many tools as I had at my disposal in order to teach the person how to undo his or her homophobia. When it came to sexism and exclusion of women, I had no patience.

My department chair was unenthusiastic about whatever I was working on, which ranged from research related to LGBT issues, to documenting sexual exploitation of patients by health professionals. The sex abuse work started through my work with the Committee on Women of the APA. My position was to advocate for women's mental health issues, and I just said, "Okay, what's going on in this country that we need to pay attention to?" I heard about all these cases of sexual exploitation by psychiatrists, and hearing these horror stories, I decided I was going to do something about it.

I decided that it was unlikely that the Committee on Women would get any educational support from the APA to do something about this unless we could document the severity or prevalence of this problem. So, we put together a questionnaire to survey the entire country about sexual exploitation of patients by health professionals, only we were not calling it exploitation then because we had to be more neutral. It was a very different world in terms of attitudes.

JGLP: The attitudes psychiatrists had about the issue of sexual contact with patients?

DR. GARTRELL: The attitude is something that we worked on for twenty years to get to where it is right now. For the purpose of neutrality, we used the term "sexual contact," as if it were just another treatment option. The Committee on Women wanted to survey psychiatrists anonymously about their attitudes regarding sex with patients, and about their own behavior. Various powers that be in the APA at that time went absolutely ballistic over that. They thought we were going to destroy the credibility of the psychiatric profession, which is a really interesting twist of logic. The committee responded that it seemed to us that it was psychiatrists who were having sexual contact with their patients—rather than those of us trying to investigate the matter—who were the ones destroying the credibility of the psychiatric profession. So they sent the committee's questionnaire through a circular, endless review process for two years in order to try to kill it. They thought they could just make it seem as though it was going to make progress, and then send it along, and that they could kind of keep me contained in that way indefinitely.

So, after a period of time I lost patience. We, my colleagues on the women's committee, my good friends Judy Herman and Sylvia Olarte, and I, said, "We're going to give you a deadline. If you can't do it by this deadline, we'll do it independently." Well, they imagined that I could not possibly get the mailing list for all the psychiatrists in the country because they controlled it. This was the era of typewriters. We didn't have the Internet. We didn't have home computers in that era. So, even though there would be a central place within the APA where they had the membership stuff—they had big mainframe computers that printed out mailing lists—

there was no way I was ever going to be able to break into those places.

I didn't have Watergate skills or anything, but I am going to tell you about some of my clandestine activities back then. In 1983, Harvard was really getting started in the continuing medical education (CME) business, and they would send out CME mailings all over the country. So I thought they must have some way of sorting mailing labels for CME courses according to different specialties. I called Harvard's CME office, and said, "I'm interested in doing a course and I wonder how I can get the labels for all the psychiatrists in the country." They said, "There's this clearinghouse in Illinois, and that's where we buy all our labels." So, I concocted a course on ethics with vague language, which referred to needing to gather data, but never really said what the specifics were. I used my own savings to buy mailing labels, which at several thousand dollars were quite costly back then, and got the labels for the entire United States. We had a questionnaire ready to go, so we just did our own envelope stuffing, got back the questionnaires, and wrote up the papers.

We submitted the first paper to APA's *American Journal of Psychiatry*. We had seven simultaneous reviewers assigned to it from day one because they were going to do everything they could to stop it. We got back reams of criticism. They didn't say "reject"; they said, "You have to modify everything." They were putting us on the path again, you know, of endless stalling. So, I didn't waste any time in responding to every single line-item. I mean, they were really idiotic criticisms. They weren't about content; they were about, "Why are you going to do this? This is going to give us a bad name." We submitted every one of those back to the journal with a cover letter saying, "By the way, if this process is not completed in a timely way, the American Psychological Association is ready to publish these data immediately." Which they were. So, the study got in, as did the other papers, and then we had a process that went on from there. Having grown up in the anti-war movement of Vietnam and learning a lot of street tactics for doing political work, those skills came in handy.

JGLP: How did you get involved in that?

DR. GARTRELL: I was in college at Stanford and it was a center of tremendous activism; you were either with us or a fascist. I chose to be in the "with us" part of that, but I was also out as a lesbian and feeling very isolated there in what was a very sexist, male-dominated political process. So it was a very welcome experience for me to start connecting with other lesbians as people started to come out in my junior and senior years of college. I had a movement that I could relate to because I felt a much stronger affinity with women.

JGLP: Did you know then that you would become a psychiatrist?

DR. GARTRELL: I actually became interested in becoming a psychiatrist about halfway through college. My major was human biology and my mentor was a psychiatrist who was very active in the American Psychiatric Association. His name was Keith Brodie, and he was president of APA at one point and then later chancellor and president at Duke. He's now retired, but then he was doing really interesting biological psychology research. I just thought it was fascinating, and I went and started working in his lab. Then he very generously agreed to sponsor whatever studies I wanted to do. He sat me down and said, "So, there are a lot of areas that need to be studied, like anything related to lesbian . . ." and I went, "Bingo! Okay." I did my first study on psychiatrists' attitudes toward lesbians and just continued on from there. He sponsored that work and helped in the next project that was related to hormones and sexual orientation. This was pre-DSM changes.

JGLP: You mean pre–deletion of homosexuality from the *Diagnostic and Statistical Manual* (DSM)?

DR. GARTRELL: Predeletion. I was interested in making it clear that homosexuality was a normal variation of sexual expression and that it was not pathological—since I had a self-interest as well as a belief system about that. In 1969 or 1970, about the time that we were doing that study, a study came out under Masters and Johnson's research team claiming that gay men had lower testosterone levels than straight men.[1] So, Dr. Brodie sponsored another study in which we measured testosterone levels in gay men at Stanford and compared them to straight men at Stanford. Our gay men had higher testosterone levels than straight men! Somehow it didn't get the kind of publicity that the other study did. I did the same study on women when I went to the National Institute of Health (NIH) as a senior medical student, and I had a lot of lesbians in DC who came out to have their blood drawn so I could look at their hormone levels. They were very primitive assays compared to what we have now. But, it was just the beginning of an era of trying to really inform people by research protocols that tried not be biased.

JGLP: It seems that early in your career you were encouraged to study subjects that might not be conventionally well received?

DR. GARTRELL: I think it was by virtue of the fact that I was a lesbian and I came out as a freshman in college. I didn't like what I saw in the world in terms of how lesbianism was handled and how people related to us as lesbians, how people related to gay men. It became a kind of strong motivator to do something about that, and since science in that era controlled social justice for us, I needed to do it through science.

JGLP: Tell me about your involvement with the gay psychiatrists.

DR. GARTRELL: I would have to say that I was the token woman on the executive committee of AGLP way back then and also the Gay and Lesbian Medical Association. The first APA meeting I went to was in 1975, and I was a junior medical student. I organized a panel, the first panel that had ever been done on lesbians at the APA. My mentor was program chair, so he helped get it on the program. I had, I think, Del Martin[2] on the panel with me and some lesbian mothers because the community back then was very focused on lesbian mother custody issues.

I remember I went to that meeting trying to find other lesbian psychiatrists or medical students—and I didn't find any. But, I could see that there were gay male psychiatrists, and somehow I met somebody that I was pretty convinced would talk to me about being gay. I said, "Do you have any meetings, or activities, or whatever?" And he said, "At the opening convocation, go up to the person who plays the organ who is a psychiatrist, and he will hand you a card, and that card will have the address to which you can go where we have a social gathering."[3]

JGLP: Wow.

DR. GARTRELL: That's how closeted everything was. So, I went to this thing. There were probably 100 men there, and I had on my big APA name badge, and I went around and I kept looking for name badges. No one had a name badge on. Finally I figured it out. That is how closeted they were—they couldn't wear name badges. So, that's how people got together for those early years when I participated, through this very circuitous route. I did my part in those various groups, and I am forgetting about my participation in the gay and lesbian task force of the APA,[4] because I was also a member of that group.

JGLP: You must have been one of the youngest people in the group, as well as being the only woman.

DR. GARTRELL: I was. I had received a Falk fellowship, where you were selected to be on a committee of the APA as a resident. I became involved in the APA as a resident, and then I was on a variety of different task forces and committees, but one of them was the gay and lesbian psychiatrists' task force. Another was supposed to be about creating a curriculum on the psychology of women and men. There'd never been such a thing in mental health training, so it was a big deal to have the APA even consider doing something about gender issues and mental health. I volunteered for the section on sexuality. A document was constructed, it was submitted, and they stopped it because of a single sentence—written by me—which was that homosexuality is a normal variation of sexual expression. The whole committee had supported that sentence and it was beyond the DSM-III decision, but they would not allow an APA publication to say that in 1981. I said, "I'm resigning from this; I'm pulling my section." All the other people who were very prominent, like Jean Baker Miller and various other people, pulled their sections too in support of this, and the document was never published. There were a lot of men working within organized psychiatry who considered my approach to things not politic enough, or too unpolished. They acted like, well, you just keep working, keep greasing the wheel, keep having conversations, and over time we'll have a greater and greater presence, greater and greater acceptability. However, I was too impatient, too young, whatever. I didn't have the time to waste doing that.

JGLP: It strikes me that you were going into this room alone, as you're describing your reception, and you're the one who had the name tag on. You seemed to have a lot of courage and poise early on.

DR. GARTRELL: Or a sort of cockiness. I don't know what it was—sort of naïveté. I mean there were times subsequently where major efforts were made to suppress me. Like, they tried to get me off the Committee on Women and put me back on a task force of gay and lesbian psychiatrists. They tried to get me out of a leadership as rapidly as possible because I was too threatening to too many people. So, there were lots of very unpleasant things that happened as well. But I feel I was really fortunate that I had a terrific support system of colleagues who, for the most part, were straight, and for the most part women, who would stand by me. I felt very honored to have been in association with such people as Jean Baker Miller, Judy Herman, and others.

JGLP: When you were sitting on the Committee of Women were you the token lesbian?

DR. GARTRELL: Yes, but I was the chair. The year that I had the greatest influence in that position I also got to select the people who were on the committee, and that happened because Keith Brodie, my mentor back then, was president of the APA and he made the appointments. I went into his office and said, "This is what I would like." We had the most diverse, the most politically progressive committee that had ever existed in the APA to that point. It was fabulous. It was a really exciting and dynamic year, and we caused a lot of trouble.

JGLP: Have you felt more affinity with women psychiatrists or women's groups than with gay psychiatrists?

DR. GARTRELL: Yes, I have. I mean it probably relates to the era in which I came out because I would go to these meetings for the Gay and Lesbian Medical Association or gay psychiatrists' groups as the only woman. I can think of one meeting for the gay psychiatrists' group that was on Fire Island. We were supposed to have an all-day meeting, but we met for about three hours, and then they had a three-hour break scheduled for them all to go out and cruise. I was like, "Wait a minute. Nobody consulted me about this. This is not my deal and this is supposed to be a business meeting." I felt marginalized a lot by those experiences.

I was going to tell you about one other thing that I did in a calm, organized way at Beth Israel because my department chair was so mad at me all the time. He kept telling me, whatever I was doing, "We are a very prestigious hospital and when your articles come out, the reporters show up. This hospital has a lot of private funding and you're going to make it difficult for us to get private funding." Well, I thought if that's the case, then I won't use my Harvard affiliation for any of my publications. That's fine. But I'm going to find it out from somebody who's not protecting his back.

So, I made an appointment to talk to the president of the hospital. I sat down with him and said, "This is what I am. This is what I do. I happen to be a lesbian, and these are the kind of research projects I do. I have been told, on a number of occasions, that I am causing difficulties for the hospital because I work in controversial areas. So, I would like to know from you, if it is the case that the kind of work that I am doing is going to be detrimental to the hospital, I will have them not put the hospital affiliation in any further publications." And he said, "I can see from what you've shown me that you're doing very reputable work. Our hospital was founded out of an interest in supporting a population that has historically been discriminated against since it is a Jewish hospital. We are not interested in promoting discrimination or limiting people's intellectual pursuits. So put your Harvard affiliation and this hospital's name on whatever you do." I had no idea that was going to happen. It was really a powerful thing.

JGLP: So affirming.

DR. GARTRELL: Yes, it was really neat. So when I experienced sexism from gay men in a small group, a leadership group, within organized psychiatry, it made me feel way more alienated than homophobia by the cultural majority.

JGLP: You probably expected more from the gay men.

DR. GARTRELL: I guess I always did.

JGLP: I want to hear about the national lesbian family study. How did you get into that area and what are your latest findings?

DR. GARTRELL: As with all my studies, they're nonfunded. This one, since it's longitudinal, I've actually gotten money for in recent years. I always work to support my research because any traditional funding sources would never, at the time that I was starting something, fund me.

We started in 1986, just before I left Boston. We wanted to study the first wave of lesbians choosing to have children by donor insemination. I was in Boston and the person I started with, Jean Hamilton, was in DC, and I was moving to California. We started advertising for participants in those two places and then added California when I got here. We gathered 154 moms. We closed the study to new participants in 1992 because there were so many big cultural changes that had already happened between 1986 and

1992 that we felt like we were getting a totally different cohort. Initially, all the people who volunteered were thinking about unknown donors because they were so terrified of having their children taken away. By the end, they were mostly going toward known donors because they wanted their children to have a known father, so among other changes that was quite visible.

We've been following them since that time, and our kids range from twelve to fifteen years old now. The interviews took place when the moms were inseminating, when they were pregnant, when their kids were one to two years old, when the kids were five, ten; we're going to do seventeen, and then when they are twenty-five. We've just interviewed the kids at ten and now we're crunching all the data. We've already established, as many people have established, that kids raised by lesbian moms are healthy, so we're not reinventing that wheel. But, we did do a Child Behavior Checklist this time, so we've got another verification of that.

However, we have found that these kids are already encountering homophobia. We ask the children in an interview about their experiences of homophobia and how those experiences relate to their experiences of racism and sexism and so on. We ask how they respond, how they feel when it happens. It's just really moving to hear the kinds of responses and the thoughtfulness, training, and preparation that these kids have had to deal with in these kinds of experiences. The kids, in addition to being very healthy, are being very thoughtfully raised to think about all "-isms," whereas if you're in a particular nonmajority group that doesn't necessarily feel motivated to think about homophobia, you might not. So, these kids are being very meaningfully educated about all those issues, which is very inspiring for our future I think.

Another finding is that the moms struggle a lot in the early years with very child-focused lives, to the exclusion of attention to their relationships, so our breakup rate is just the same as heterosexual relationships. Everybody was hoping to see that lesbian moms would do it better. My advice to people from what I have learned is to be more attentive to their relationships. You cannot just not want it for ten years, and then kind of look over, and say, "By the way, we haven't had sex for ten years," or "Why were you out for three nights with someone else?"

I have often said about the lesbian family studies that, if I were a mom in the study, it wouldn't have continued as long as it has. That is because it would be awfully difficult to do the study and be a really devoted parent. If you're going to do something longitudinal, you kind of need to have that space in your life.

The lesbian family study is a big job. It's a descriptive study, although we do throw small bones to those who are desperate for us to quantify something, but it's really not about that. Now, there are lots of people who want to do research on lesbian families and there are going to be lots of opportunities for people to do highly controlled studies. We're doing a different kind.

JGLP: But it's that longitudinal view that makes it so unique and wonderful to really get a look at the children's and parents' lives.

DR. GARTRELL: That's what we think.

JGLP: It is still hard to get funding for studies having to do with sexuality, and one hears from people who are doing research that they have to carefully word grant requests to avoid controversial phrases. But I guess there's a freedom in doing research independently, although it's a hard road to take.

DR. GARTRELL: There is. Sometimes I've thought, "Wouldn't my life be so easy if I got a huge amount of money to carry the study forward." But, there is a tremendous usefulness in feeling that my energy for spending thousands of hours applying, documenting, reporting can be used to actually do the research.

I have always set my life up so that my week is very varied. I have my clinical part of the week in the first half and my research in the second half. When I was teaching regularly, that was in there as well. To me, it has felt like a really nice way of always staying interested in what I'm doing because it changes even as the week evolves.

JGLP: You and Dee Mosbacher[5] have been together for a long time. How did you meet?

DR. GARTRELL: Well, as a senior medical student I went to work at NIH in neurology for six months, so I moved to Washington, DC. I had met Joan Biren[6] through a friend out here, and she found me a place to live in a house in DC, and Dee was one of the people who lived in the house. I met Dee when I was asked to go to the airport and pick up "a lesbian with blond streaked hair" who would be getting off the plane from Houston.

We became involved in 1975, and we've been together now twenty-eight years. We've just been a lot of places since then. She applied to graduate school, got a PhD in psychology, and then she decided to go to medical school. When she got into medical school at Baylor, I was in a terrible conflict about going to Houston with her because I didn't want to work down there. I was really excited about the work I was doing in Boston. I moved to Texas with her and got a faculty position at the University of Texas. However, the second day I was there, the vice chair of the psychiatry department told a patient her diagnosis was that she was a "hysterical cunt." I decided that day I was going back to Boston, despite how much I loved Dee and valued our relationship. So, I went back and commuted while Dee stayed in Houston in medical school, and then she came to Cambridge Hospital to do her residency. Then we were back where we've been, basically, in the same place ever since. When she finished her residency, we made the move we had always planned to San Francisco. We fly our rainbow flag without fear and live in all the beauty that this city has to offer. I feel very privileged and fortunate to live here. We don't have children; our dependents are two Maltese dogs.

JGLP: I'm impressed with how you've always been out there with topics and missions that are really cutting-edge, that you're not afraid to put your ideas out and deal with whatever consequences.

DR. GARTRELL: Well, there have been difficult times. But I feel like I've succeeded more than I've failed—even if the success has taken more than a decade in some of the areas in which I've worked. I feel very fortunate to have had, so far in life, a lot of meaningful challenges that I've been able to do my best to face. I hope that continues.

JGLP: We hope so too.

NOTES

1. See Kolodny, R. C., Masters, W. H., Hendryx, J. & Toro, G. (1971), Plasma testosterone and semen analysis in male homosexuals. *New England Journal of Medicine,* 285:1170-1174; and Kolodny, R. C., Jacobs, L. S., Masters, W. H.,

Toro, G. & Daughaday, W. H. (1972), Plasma gonadotrophins and prolactin in male homosexuals. *Lancet,* 2:18-20.

2. Del Martin was a founder of the Daughters of Bilitis, an early homophile organization.

3. That organist was the late John Fryer, MD. See David Scasta's article on John E. Fryer, MD, and the Dr. H. Anonymous episode, Chapter 1 in this book.

4. The predecessor to what is today the APA's Committee on Gay, Lesbian, and Bisexual Issues.

5. Dr. Gartrell's partner, Dee Mosbacher, MD, is a psychiatrist and Academy Award–nominated filmmaker who produces documentary films on homophobia.

6. Joan Biren (JEB) is a lesbian photographer known for her photographs of lesbians and lesbian life.

SELECTED BIBLIOGRAPHY

Journal Articles

Brodie, H. K. H., Gartrell, N., Rhue, T. & Doering, C. (1974), Plasma testosterone levels in heterosexual and homosexual men. *Amer. J. Psychiatry,* 131(1):82-83.

Gartrell, N., Brodie, H. K. H. & Kraemer, H. (1974), Psychiatrists' attitudes toward female homosexuality. *J. Nerv. & Ment. Dis.,* 159(2):141-144.

Gartrell, N., Chase, T. & Loriaux, L. (1977), Plasma testosterone levels in heterosexual and homosexual women. *Amer. J. Psychiatry,* 134(10):1117-1119.

Gartrell, N. (1981), The lesbian as a single woman. *Amer. J. Psychotherapy,* 35(4): 502-516.

Gartrell, N. (1984), Combating homophobia in the psychotherapy of lesbians. *Women Ther.,* 3(1):13-29.

Gartrell, N., Herman, J., Olarte, S., Feldstein, M. & Localio, R. (1986), Psychiatrist-patient sexual contact: Results of a national survey. I. Prevalence. *Amer. J. Psychiatry,* 143(9):1126-1131.

Herman, J., Gartrell, N., Olarte, S., Feldstein, M. & Localio, R. (1987), Psychiatrist-patient sexual contact: Results of a national survey. II. Attitudes. *Amer. J. Psychiatry,* 144(2):164-169.

Gartrell, N., Herman, J., Olarte, S., Feldstein, M. & Localio, R. (1987), Reporting practices of psychiatrists who knew of sexual misconduct by colleagues. *Amer. J. Orthopsychiat.,* 57(2):287-295.

Gartrell, N., Herman, J., Olarte, S., Feldstein, M. & Localio, R. (1988), Management and rehabilitation of sexually exploitative therapists. *Hosp. & Comm. Psychiat.,* 39(10):1070-1074.

Gartrell, N., Herman, J., Olarte, S., Feldstein, M. & Localio, R. (1988), Sexual contact between psychiatric residents and educators: Results of a national survey. *Amer. J. Psychiatry,* 145(6):690-694.

Gartrell, N. (1992), Boundaries in lesbian therapy relationships. *Women Ther.,* 12(3): 29-50.

Gartrell, N., Milliken, N., Goodson, W. H., Thiemann, S. & Lo, B. (1992), Physician-patient sexual contact: Prevalence and problems. *West. J. Med.,* 157(2): 139-143.

Gartrell, N. & Sanderson, B. (1994), Sexual abuse of women by women in counseling, therapy, and advocacy. *Women Ther.,* 15(1):39-54.

Banks, A. & Gartrell, N. (1995), Hormones and sexual orientation—A questionable link. *J. Homosex.,* 27(3/4):247-268.

Gartrell, N., Hamilton, J., Banks, A., Mosbacher, D., Reed, N., Sparks, C. & Bishop, H. (1996), The national lesbian family study I: Interviews with prospective mothers. *Amer. J. Orthopsychiat.,* 66(2):272-281.

Gartrell, N., Banks, A., Hamilton, J., Reed, N., Bishop, H. & Rodas, C. (1999), The national lesbian family study II: Interviews of mothers with toddlers. *Amer. J. Orthopsychiat.,* 69(3):362-369.

Gartrell, N., Banks, A., Reed, N., Hamilton, J., Rodas, C. & Deck, A. (2000), The national lesbian family study III: Interviews of mothers of five-year-olds. *Amer. J. Orthopsychiat.,* 70(4):542-548.

Book Chapters

Gartrell, N. (1982), Hormones and homosexuality. In: *Homosexuality: Social, Psychological, and Biological Issues,* ed. W. Paul, J. D. Weinrich, J. C. Gonsiorek & M. E. Hotredt. Beverly Hills: Sage Publications, pp. 169-182.

Gartrell, N. (1982), Sexual problems in gay patients. In: *Treatment Interventions in Human Sexuality,* ed. C. Nadelson & D. Marcott. New York: Plenum, pp. 395-410.

Gartrell, N., Olarte, S. & Herman, J. (1986), Institutional resistance to self-study: A case report. In: *Sexual Exploitation of Patients by Health Professionals,* ed. A. Burgess. Philadelphia: Praeger, pp. 285-300.

Gartrell, N., Herman, J., Olarte, S., Feldstein, M. & Localio, R. (1989), Prevalence of psychiatrist-patient sexual contact. In: *Sexual Exploitation in Professional Relationships,* ed. G. Gabbard. Washington, DC: American Psychiatric Press, pp. 3-14.

Gartrell, N. (1994), Boundaries in lesbian therapist-client relationships. In: *Lesbian and Gay Psychology: Theory, Research, and Clinical Applications,* ed. B. Greene & G. Herek. Thousand Oaks, CA: Sage Publications, pp. 98-117.

Gartrell, N. (1995), Lesbian feminist fights organized psychiatry. In: *Feminist Foremothers in Women's Studies, Psychology, and Mental Health,* ed. P. Chesler, E. D. Rothblum & E. Cole. Binghamton, NY: Harrington Park Press, pp. 205-212.

Gartrell, N., Milliken, N., Goodson III, H., Thiemann, S. & Lo, B. (1995), Physician-patient sexual contact: Prevalence and problems. In: *Breach of Trust: Sexual Exploitations by Health Care Professionals and Clergy,* ed. J. C. Gonsiorek. Thousand Oaks, CA: Sage Publications, pp. 18-28.

Banks, A. & Gartrell, N. (1996), Lesbians in the medical setting. In: *Textbook of Homosexuality and Mental Health,* ed. R. P. Cabaj & T. Stein. Washington, DC: American Psychiatric Press, pp. 659-672.

Gartrell, N. (1997), Out in academic psychiatry. In: *Lesbians in Academia,* ed. B. Mintz & E. D. Rothblum. New York: Routledge, pp. 63-68.

Gartrell, N. (2000), Swimming upstream: Voyage of a lesbian psychiatrist. In: *Psychotherapy at the Millennium: Personal Visions,* ed. J. Shay & J. Wheelis. New York: Irvington Publishers, pp. 126-146.

Books

Gartrell, N. (1994), *Bringing Ethics Alive: Feminist Ethics in Psychotherapy Practice.* Binghamton, NY: The Haworth Press.

Gartrell, N. & Rothblum, E. D. (2001), *Everyday Mutinies: Funding Lesbian Activism.* Binghamton, NY: The Haworth Press.

Chapter 10

An Interview with Stuart E. Nichols, MD

Kenn Ashley

Stuart E. Nichols received his BA in 1957 from the Virginia Military Institute. He obtained his medical degree from the Medical College of Virginia in 1961. He completed his internship at Letterman General Hospital in San Francisco in 1962. He did his psychiatric residency training at Manhattan State Hospital between 1964 and 1967.

His professional career included serving as Clinical Director of the Drug Addiction Research Unit and Assistant Director of the Division of Narcotics for the New York State Department of Health (1967-1968). He went on to become the Director of Psychiatry (Addiction Services) for the NYC Community Mental Health Board (NYCCMHB) while simultaneously holding the position of Director of Psychiatry (Corrections) and Acting First Deputy Commissioner for the NYCCMHB (1968-1970). He served as Director of the Cumberland Methadone Maintenance Treatment Program (MMTP) of Beth Israel Medical Center (BIMC) in NYC (1970-1971), Director of Addiction Services at Gracie Square Hospital (1971-1973), and then Unit Director for the MMTP of BIMC (1973-1975). From 1975 to 1976, he was Chief of BIMC's Drug Detoxification Service and in 1976 became Associate Chief of the Medical and Psychiatric Services of BIMC's MMTP. He later went on to become Medical Director of that service.

This chapter appeared originally under the same title in *Journal of Gay & Lesbian Psychotherapy* 6(4):55-71.

American Psychiatry and Homosexuality: An Oral History
Published by The Haworth Press, Inc., 2007.
doi:10.1300/6049_11

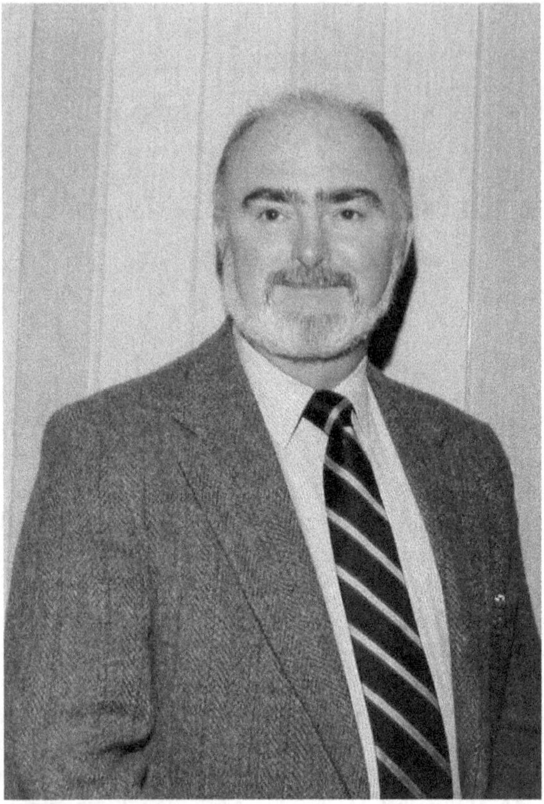

Dr. Nichols was also an Associate Professor of Psychiatry at Mount Sinai Hospital and Medical Center in New York City before his retirement. He was a member of the Group for the Advancement of Psychiatry (Committee on Human Sexuality). He was a founding member of Gay Psychiatrists of New York (GPNY) in 1978 and its first President from 1978 to 1980. He was a founding member of both the American Association of Physicians for Human Rights (now known as the Gay and Lesbian Medical Association) and the New York Physicians for Human Rights. He was President of the Association of Gay and Lesbian Psychiatrists (AGLP) from 1983 to 1984.

Dr. Nichols was a Fellow of the American Psychiatric Association and served on numerous APA committees and components, at both the national and New York County District Branch (NYCDB) level.

He chaired the APA's Ad Hoc Committee on AIDS (later the Commission on AIDS), was a member of the APA's Committee on Gay, Lesbian, and Bisexual Issues, and a Deputy Assembly Representative for the GLB Caucus of the APA. He chaired the NYCDB's Committee on GLB Issues as well, was elected to serve on the NYCDB's Council, and was serving as NYCDB President when he had a disabling stroke in 1994.

The cognitive defects he suffered from his stroke made it difficult for Dr. Nichols to remember specific dates and names in this interview, which took place a few months before his untimely death in June 2002. He began by talking about his reluctance to be interviewed.

DR. NICHOLS: When I was asked to do this interview a while back, I did not feel able to do it. But after Bert Schaffner was interviewed,[1] I got a copy of that and I slowly read it. I was so impressed, and it brought back a lot of memories of my early days before I came out and all that; and it motivated me to at least try and do this interview.

JGLP: I understand you were active in the formation of gay psychiatrists' groups at both the local and national levels.

DR. NICHOLS: Well, let me start with my childhood and lead into that because with me it all ties in together. I grew up down in Virginia, was raised Catholic, and started in high school to have sexual feelings toward other boys. I remember I was open about that. I remember groups of guys would get around and they would start talking about how girls turned them on and how they got erections; and I would say that never happened to me. I was very open and I remember at some point saying, "Well, maybe I'm queer." It was the word we used in those days. They all reassured me, "Oh no, not you," and that essentially taught me to shut up and to keep those thoughts to myself. I learned to do that.

Another big influence was being raised Catholic—fairly strictly and devout—and being taught in Catholic school through high school, by the nuns and the monks, that homosexuality was a sin—that people might be tempted that way, but it was a testing from God, something to which you should not succumb. If you wanted to be saved, you resisted it, and not only would you go to heaven, but you would also live a more fulfilling life. If you gave into it, all hell would break loose.

Also, as a young boy, I did not know any gay men, except for one disgusting old man, as I called him. I wouldn't call him so old these days. He would hang around the tennis courts where I used to go play because they had a public toilet and he was obviously there trying to pick up boys. He was really a very disagreeable person, and so, combined with the church teachings and even the rejection from my classmates, I thought if I did succumb to my homosexual feelings, that I would turn out like that man. I still had the feelings, but I resisted acting out on them all the way through medical school. I went for my internship, believe it or not, in San Francisco.

JGLP: Fortuitous, it seems.

DR. NICHOLS: Fortuitous, yes. But when I got there, there was a young woman named Eleanor whom I'd known in Richmond. She had been going out with one of my best friends from medical school. They had broken up and she had flown to San Francisco to work and I started dating her. In fact, I kind of proposed to her, but I admitted to her that I had a sexual problem. If I got too close to women, I really lost interest. She was smart enough to suggest to me that I could be homosexual. Well, I broke up with her right away. Also, her former boyfriend from Virginia, when he learned that she and I were going together, renewed his interest and proposed to her, so she flew back and they married and had children and grandchildren; in fact, I'm going to visit them this week.

I went to San Francisco shortly after Eleanor flew back to Virginia. A guy I was interning with wanted to show me this crazy bar, which turned out to be a gay bar, and we went there. It was not just a gay bar; it was a really crazy one with all kinds of people—I mean hustlers and street people, a mixture of all kinds of people. And I couldn't believe that some of these, especially the more normal-looking types, were homosexual because my idea up to that point was that homosexuals were all dirty old men. I asked one of the normal-looking guys if I could talk with him. I explained I was a doctor and that I just wanted to learn more about this. So he agreed to meet and we talked; we ended up after a few meetings having sex. I thought, "This is the only time I'm going to do it, so I might as well see what if feels like." But when I actually had sex with him I realized, "Oh my God! This feels more real. I am homosexual." I had to accept what I had been denying for so many years. Also around that time, I met a young man named Phil living in San

Francisco and started dating. We became lovers very quickly. My internship ended in 1962 and I had to go to boot camp because I was in the army. I was stationed in San Francisco by the army.

JGLP: Where were you stationed in the military?

DR. NICHOLS: After boot camp, I was with the Special Forces and I was in Badtolz, which is in Bavaria—it's a tiny little town. So Phil agreed to fly over. He quit his job and we had a very romantic, idealistic Christmas together. During this time, while he was there, I got the news that I was being transferred to Berlin. So I went there and again I was assigned to some medical unit there. I was only in Berlin for about a month when Phil joined me. He had decided that he was going to stay in Europe and try and find a job and we were going to live happily ever after.

One day, when I was about to go to lunch, two men came into the office. "Captain Nichols?" they asked. "Yes." "We need to speak to you for a moment." They came in and they accused me of being homosexual. At first, I tried to deny it. They had a document in front of them which indicated that they had been following me for the last several weeks. They had every place I'd been, including some gay bars. And I realized, as they were talking, they were men I had seen around, just knew in Berlin. Anyway, they said, "Look, if you are homosexual, just tell us. It will be the best for the army and the best for you. We'll just separate, you know, no problems."

I thought about it. I tried to forestall it, but then I said, "You know that's right. I have just accepted that I am gay. I really don't belong in the army." So I admitted it. Well, they placed me under arrest. The army's position at that time was that when a homosexual was found, the person had to be transferred to another base within twenty-four hours. Supposedly, the other soldiers would be so horrified if they knew, that they might kill you or who knows what. I was put on a night train out of Berlin and sent to Munich.

I'm making this a long story, but the strange part of this is that I was the only person allowed to be on that car, with a guard at each end. Through the middle of the night, I didn't sleep much. I got to Berlin the next morning and waited there in my seat in the railroad car for the military police to come get me. They didn't come. Eventually the train seemed about ready to leave again, so I picked up my bags and got off and waited in the station. Nobody came. Eventually I found my way to the hospital. I knew that I was going to report to the commanding officer, who was a doctor. He welcomed me and arranged to get me settled in a room in the bachelors'/officers' quarters.

It's kind of a funny—I went through this whole processing for this new post in Munich. It took almost all day; they assigned me quarters, etc. By the end of that day, I went to my room, closed the door, and for the first time I really had time to react to what had happened. I started thinking about my family, coming home to Virginia, and my parents learning about all that had happened. I really was considering suicide; it felt that it was probably the easiest way out, the least messy. And just as I was thinking this, there was a knock on my door. I opened it and there was this gorgeous man with just a little towel wrapped around his waist, saying, "Hi, I'm your roommate"; there were two V-shaped bedrooms off the end of the hall. I thought, "Yeah, sure. You think I'm going to fall for this? I'm not that stupid." Actually, that was the first thing that got me resisting what was happening to me. It turned out he wasn't gay; he wasn't trying to seduce me. What he was asking was if I would let his girlfriend in—who was coming to illegally spend the night with him—because he was going to go take a shower. I said, "Sure." That's kind of the end of that story! The point is that the experience got me to come out of my depression and to start fighting to survive.

I expected to be in Munich only a few days, but instead I was there for three or four months. I was assigned a position in the outpatient clinic and nothing was ever explained to me; I just worked there. Then one day I was called in and told, "You're going back to the States to be discharged." I got my things together and flew back to a post on the East Coast. I think I was to be there just overnight and the next morning I was going to get the official discharge papers. I'd also been told, when I had first been confronted after my admission of homosexuality, that I was going to be dishonorably discharged and that I would lose my medical license. All these bad things were going to happen. When I was waiting there for discharge, I called the Judge Advocate lawyers and said I wished to remain anonymous, but could I speak to a lawyer about my discharge. I was given someone's name and I explained to him what was happening. This guy said he didn't really know much about this issue, but if I could call him back in a day or two, he would find out as much as he could and give me the best advice on it. What he eventually told me was that my situation fell into a murky area. He said it was not clear that I would be discharged, but he advised me that, if I retained my license, I should not work in an area where I would be very noticeable or visible; that I was not to make waves and that I should stay in the background. I said, "Okay." And actually, that's one of the main reasons I chose to work in drug addiction—nobody wanted to work in drug addiction back then and nobody cared.

So now that I was back in the States, one of the first things I did was go see an old psychiatry professor of mine from medical school who was then living in New York. I told him what had happened, and his advice to me was, "Well, you have to be cured." He said one could only get a good psychoanalysis in three places, and since one of those places was New York, I decided I might as well stay there. He picked out a guy for me whom I saw four days a week for about three years. I failed miserably. However, it really helped in that I did get more in touch with my feelings and how strong they were. I got to know myself better.

Also, while I was in psychoanalysis, I decided to become a psychiatrist, and following the advice I got in the Army, I went to a place where nobody would notice very much: Manhattan General Hospital on Wards Island. I did my residency there, and in my third year of residency, I worked on their drug addiction unit. I then went on to stay in that field. The problem I had is that people wanted to promote me and it was a little difficult to stay in the background. I later went to New York's Beth Israel Medical Center where I ran a detoxification ward. One day, a patient under my care came to me crying in a really distressed state. He was a Hispanic man, a very butch muscular guy, who told me he'd just found out that he was gay—or whatever he called it. I panicked. I was kind of cold to him. I wasn't warm and I wasn't really reassuring to him. I was frightened, wondering, "Oh my God! Is he going to pick up that I'm gay also?" Well, two days later, I heard he'd committed suicide. That was a big influence on my life because I really felt, in part, responsible. I did not do what I could have done. He was in distress, needed help, and I withheld it. I didn't have to tell him I was gay. I just had not been sympathetic. I think that made me resolve never to consider the danger to me. That changed me and started me on the path to being more open about myself.

JGLP: What about that path?

DR. NICHOLS: Okay, let's go into the gay activities. I'd become a psychiatrist. I joined the APA and I started going to the annual meetings. I forget where the first one I went to was, but after the day's meetings had ended, I went to a bar—a gay bar—and had a drink. The guy next to me just happened to say, "Oh, you're not from here. What brings you to town?" And I just opened up and told him, "Well, I'm a psychiatrist and I'm here for the meetings." He said, "Oh, really?" Then the guy next to him said, "I'm a psychiatrist too." It turned out that almost half the people around the bar were gay psychiatrists. That totally floored all of us because within the profession we'd been so hidden—to strangers anyway. So we called ourselves the Gay-P-A, and we agreed each year that at the annual meeting we would pick a particular day and a particular bar and meet there. That went on for several years and I made some good friends.

In 1970, the Gay Activists Alliance (GAA) zapped an APA annual meeting in San Francisco and disrupted it.[2] In the middle of a scientific meeting, this bunch of crazy men came in and disrupted the proceedings and said they were not going to allow the psychiatrists to continue unless there was a change in the APA position on homosexuality and unless homosexuals were treated differently. They would not let the meeting go on. Eventually a compromise was reached—the activists agreed to leave and the APA, at its next annual meeting,[3] would have a presentation on homosexuality giving various points of view. Then, at the following meeting,[4] there was a psychiatrist in disguise who spoke as openly homosexual. He was in a total body costume. That man was John Fryer of Pennsylvania, a good friend of mine.[5] That was another part of the history of the early coming out of the APA and of its dealings with the issue of homosexuality.

After a few years, the gay psychiatrists who would eventually form AGLP had become more organized and they didn't want to just have a social meeting. There was a meeting held away from the convention premises. It was announced in the APA program book that tells what's happening that there was a meeting for gay psychiatrists. I saw that notice and I really had mixed feelings. I was scared to attend; I wanted to attend. I remember going to that hotel and walking past the door a couple of times, trying to look in and see who was there, and eventually I went in. By the end of the meeting, I was really happy to have been there. I really felt supported. When we were leaving, I introduced myself to someone from New York whose name I can't remember. I told him I was from New York and that if I could be of any help during the year to let me know. And I started coming out that way. After a few years, the group slowly became more and more visible. In fact, I think they agreed to take one of the exhibition booths at the convention center and to show themselves. I remember the title of the booth was "Gay Love: Good Medicine." Most of the psychiatrists walked by that booth, kind of looking at it; very few people came in. But we were just being there and being open. Some gay people later told me that it was very reassuring that you could be that open and not be burned at the stake.

JGLP: Was the booth focusing on gay love or gay psychiatrists?

DR. NICHOLS: I really don't remember, but I think it was more that there is nothing wrong with gay love; that gay love is just as good as nongay love. They showed a picture of a couple holding hands, Emery Hetrick, who was a psychiatrist, and his lover Damien Martin.[6] It was an eye-opener for many people.

One of the things that the group proposed was that since the APA at that time had created other minority caucuses, that the gay psychiatrists should become an official minority group. Well, this threw the APA Assembly into an uproar and they just couldn't handle it. Instead, they referred the issue back to each district branch (DB) to advise them on the matter, and they would meet again a year later. During that year, the APA was divided into eastern and western parts. I was in charge of the east and Jim Krajeski was in charge of the west. The two of us visited as many district branches as we could, meeting with the executive committees of the DBs when they were deciding that issue. This was pretty strenuous. By the time the APA met the following year, a number of district branches, perhaps a majority, had agreed that we had a reasonable proposition and that we should be granted minority status. We were clearly treated as minorities. The individual who was then president of the APA called for a voice vote and very quickly said, "The ayes have it" and slammed his gavel down. The people who were really opposed to it started saying that it was a quick vote, and he said, "The vote is closed. You had your chance." That's the end of that story, but that's how that got started.

JGLP: When did GPNY, now GLPNY, the New York gay psychiatrists' group begin and what was your involvement with that?

DR. NICHOLS: That also grew out of a meeting, I believe, in San Francisco where David Kessler, who was the chair of a local gay psychiatrist's group, hosted a session during the annual meeting. He was discussing how the SF group got formed and what the results had been. Again, I went to attend it, but I was very hesitant—who knew who was going to be there? I was trying to look around and see if there was anyone I knew there before I went in. But, I went in and sat down, and who knows but right across the aisle from me was Emery Hetrick, another psychiatrist from Beth Israel. At first I panicked, but I couldn't get up and run out. Then I realized if he's in the meeting, he's probably not a foe.

JGLP: So until then you had not known about Emery?

DR. NICHOLS: I knew Emery because we were both in the Psychiatry Department—I knew him from grand rounds, that sort of thing. I had no idea he was gay. After that meeting, Emery and I met outside and said that it had been wonderful and decided to start a similar gay psychiatrists' group in New York.[7] We came back and—between Emery and myself—we knew a number of people who were gay, or we thought were gay. We sent them an invitation saying we were organizing a meeting for this organization and gave them a date. Amazingly, nine people showed up at that first meeting. Very nervous at first, everybody kind of looking over their shoulder, but that was the first meeting and the beginning of the gay psychiatric group in New York. It's been going on ever since then.

During the first year we had to choose a name, and one of the members objected to the word "gay" being in the name, so we became the New York Physicians for Human Rights.[8] Then that person never came to another meeting. So the name was changed shortly thereafter to Gay Psychiatrists of New York and then Gay and Lesbian Psychiatrists of New York a few years later. It has gone through its changes but has continued to meet ever since. Bert Schaffner joined the group near the end of the first year. What happened also to the group is that it started growing, getting so large that we had at times to split into two groups. We were meeting in Bert's apartment, as everything does,[9] and with fifty to sixty people showing up for a meeting, half of them would meet in Bert's living space and the other half would meet in the area where he sees patients.

JGLP: What kinds of topics were discussed?

DR. NICHOLS: There was no stated topic. People were just there to share. During those early days, there was always someone who was just coming out. Bert and I also had a part in forming a general medical group for all doctors.[10] They were organized, again, in Bert's apartment. At that meeting AIDS was a fairly new phenomenon. It wasn't even called AIDS.

JGLP: GRID[11] probably.

DR. NICHOLS: GRID—you're right. At the end of the meeting, I asked a couple of the internists who was it that was providing emotional support for these patients. They looked at each other and then said that they guessed that I was. I told them I did not do that kind of work, but they said since I was the first one to ask the question, I should try it. I did start a meeting for HIV patients for a mixed group of people. The outlook for their lives, for their longevity, was bleak at that point. So it became a very supportive group.

JGLP: Were they all physicians? At some point I know that you started a group for HIV-infected physicians.

DR. NICHOLS: I'm going to get to that next. This one was not just a group for physicians. This group was for anyone. Eventually that group was taken over by a physician member of the group when I chose to leave it. He led it for a while, then it became part of GMHC,[12] although I'm not sure how. Also, a female doctor I'd known came to me after finding out she had been infected with HIV by a needle stick. She had looked around for support groups for women but couldn't find any that weren't for drug addicts. She asked me if I would help her try and form such a group for non-addicted women. We sent around a letter to doctors treating AIDS patients and got a few names. We started to meet, and I thought that once it formed, I would no longer be a part of it. I was told that I was one of the leaders, so for a number of years I also helped run that group.

JGLP: That was a group for HIV-infected women doctors?

DR. NICHOLS: Actually, any woman. No one was turned away from the group. They did not have to be a doctor or whatever, but it was mostly for women who couldn't find people on their level to talk to. In fact, one of the first women was the wife of an HIV patient; she herself was not infected. That went on for a number of years.

I had, during this time, started trying to form a group for the doctors treating AIDS. A few would come, but somehow it never gelled, so I gave that up. Later one of those doctors approached me to meet with a few doctors; there were four of them. One of the doctors who treats a lot of AIDS patients called me and asked if I would try again to form a group for physicians with AIDS. He had a couple of patients and he knew several other internists who were also treating doctors with AIDS. I agreed and we started the doctors' group. That was right at the time when doctors who were infected were being threatened with the loss of their medical license. That group grew very rapidly and that's the one that expanded so much. Doctors would even come from Pennsylvania to attend the group because there was nothing like it anywhere else. That group started more than twenty years ago and it is still meeting. It's a much smaller group now, with four to six doctors. Since treatment is available for HIV, it's obviously changed the character of the meetings. Bert and I run the group in his apartment. We meet twice a month, every other week.

JGLP: From your perspective, what are the most important changes in working with physicians with HIV?

DR. NICHOLS: Obviously, the most important change is the availability now of effective treatments. It's no longer something that's going to kill you in a short period of time. In fact, we have a member in the group who almost died of AIDS. He had to drop out of the group because he was so sick. Effective treatment became available at just about that time and now he has rejoined the group. We heard from doctors who foolishly gave up their medical license back in the early days when doctors were being scapegoated. I know of one who has never been sick but who voluntarily gave up his medical license and can no longer practice medicine.

JGLP: They were threatening to take doctors' licenses away or were they actually taking away licenses?

DR. NICHOLS: Well, they were threatening to. The doctors were considered pariahs. They were treated as if *they* were the problem.

That *they* were passing AIDS on to patients. Hysteria, of course, but that was the climate of the time. There was no effective treatment, so AIDS meant you weren't going to live very long and that you would have a pretty horrible death.

JGLP: You said there was thought of ending the group.

DR. NICHOLS: Because the group is dwindling; actually we met this week and we had one person there. Two members had reasons they weren't there, but it is getting so small. Also, there is the fact of effective treatments—now that AIDS is not an immediate death sentence, is the group needed? We found a lot of people would come for eight to eighteen months, would get from it what they needed, and then they would drop out. We asked ourselves if the group was really necessary. Four or five people said that they really needed it, so we've continued it. Bert and I are group participants as much as the AIDS patients are at this point. I, with my near-death experiences, and with Bert getting older, we all have something to contribute. It's helpful.

Which brings me to my stroke. I was flying so high and doing so much, involved in so many things. I was just beginning my term as President of the New York County District Branch when I had my stroke. In fact, when I gave my presidential address, I was making no sense. I'd been busy doing so many things and this was suddenly stopped, cut short. I have a report of some test that was done the first few months after my stroke. I couldn't name an object—a pencil—held in front of me; really, I was severely limited. I've slowly come back more and more, daring to start to function again. This interview is an example of that. The other thing I realize, as I've had this rebirth—if you want to call it that—is how pushy I was. Given the way I came out in the army and all, I was so frightened, although I didn't feel that way. I was very pushy. I wanted to do things but it was hard for me to cooperate with people. Bert can tell you about that. As Bert and I started some of these groups, I was limited in my perspective and not always for the best, of course. Since I've had the stroke I can see the way I used to function. Yes, I accomplished things that I'm proud of—I'm not taking that back. But I was very fortunate to hook up with Bert. Bert was able to soften my approach. Bert is very . . . I can't find the words.

JGLP: Bert is very thoughtful, good at synthesizing things, seeing the broader picture, and a good mediator.

DR. NICHOLS: Exactly! Whereas I was really stuck and very sharp and forceful. The things I was trying to do were good things, but the way I was approaching it or approaching people wasn't always the best. Bert and I were a good combination because I think I had the guts to take steps. I really attribute that to my early experience of getting kicked out of the army and all those things. I decided that if I was going to function, I just had to go for broke. It also made me unable to soften and really listen to other people's points of view. I really had to go for it and sink or swim. Bert and my combining to do things was really good because I would come up with an idea and it might be off the wall. Bert would just let it pass, but he would bring the group around. We were a very good combination. I'm not putting myself down. I think to open new doors, if you put it that way, perhaps you needed someone like me to do that. Fortunately I had someone like Bert with me to smooth over the rough edges. I think we accomplished a lot together that neither one of us would have probably done alone.

I also need to give credit to Pete. Pete Garcia and I have been together for twenty-six years. I met him at a time when a lot of these things I became involved with were just starting. I was very tentative and laid-back. Pete, on the other hand, had come out as a very young man living in Spanish Harlem. He had to accept very early that he was gay. This meant to him that he was going to have to wear a dress or something—that was his image of what gay people were! He'd been active very early in the GAA, later the National Gay and Lesbian Task Force. In fact, they asked him to form a gay Hispanic section. When he and I got together, I was taking baby steps, careful steps in doing some of these things. He was challenging me, asking me what I was afraid of, asking me why I didn't go for it. I'm so lucky that he was around because he helped me to become more open and active, to do things that I probably wouldn't have done if I hadn't had that gentle push by my side. He's an important person in the development of whatever I became.

JGLP: You've also had some serious medical challenges.

DR. NICHOLS: I've had four near-death experiences. During the last one, I had bypass surgery on some arteries in my brain. I was on the heart-lung machine. I was asleep during the procedure, but I was awake shortly thereafter. It's the first near-death experience I've had where I was really aware of it shortly after it happened, of how impaired I was. All the other near-death experiences—my heart or my stroke—it was weeks, months after before I really knew what was happening. I was alive, but I was really out of it. With this one, the afternoon of the surgery, they brought Pete in to see me and he freaked out seeing all of the tubes. I was aware of what was happening. That's the real difference. This was pretty immediate, and that's what struck me.

That's really been good for me, which is why I agreed to do this interview. It was important for me to at least try, even if I flubbed it. That experience made me recognize that we all have a limited time in life. If you want to do things, take the chance. Do it now because you may not be here tomorrow. I feel so much better having come to that point. I was really in the doldrums for the last whatever years—not daring to do very much. I've always, since I came out of hiding as a gay man, dared to do things. I lost that for a while after I got sick, until six months ago. I really feel good, as I say, coming alive again. I'm the old me, limited but living life much more the way I used to during most of my years.

JGLP: With your perspective on the gay civil rights movement, what have been the most striking changes over time?

DR. NICHOLS: This is not quite answering your question, but one of the reasons I wanted to do this interview is because the young gay and lesbian people today are just so comfortable and so unaware of how difficult it was to get where we are. I think that's a danger because if you don't know your history, you're doomed to relive it. It's really not that many years ago. It scares me that people are so comfortable.

JGLP: I agree. Even though I came out when things were much easier, I wonder if the youth of today would have the courage, the commitment, to face the challenges of those who fought for the civil rights so many people now take for granted.

DR. NICHOLS: I remember in high school my mother said that she thought "separate but equal" was entirely fair. I challenged her, even though it was the way things were in Virginia at that time. I was different—I don't know why. I attribute my sexuality, my being different there, to giving me an ability not to just accept the pabulum that was being presented. It gave me my ability to question things. I'm amazed that it started that early, but I was different too.

JGLP: I remember other things that seemed very important to you—gardening and the fish pond at your place in New Jersey.

DR. NICHOLS: Yes, those were things I was doing before my stroke. I was really spread too thin. I was into antiques, the fish pond. Oh! I did not tell you an important thing. When I was twenty, a friend suggested that I get a general physical. Amazingly, when they drew my blood, it came out looking like milk. I went through an extensive work-up, all sorts of tests were run, but not much was known about cholesterol at that time. The result was they could not tell me what was wrong but the internist's final words to me were, "If you want to accomplish something in your life, start now." Fortunately, my blood condition cleared up for many years. This experience was important to me because at an early age I was told that I probably would not live an extensive life. That helped me take risks that I otherwise would not have probably taken.

Let me tell you about when I remet the psychoanalyst who tried to cure me of being gay. At the APA annual meeting when we were lobbying for minority status, my old analyst was an assembly representative from New York. Not only that, he'd been in medical school with one of the other gay psychiatrists—I think it was David Kessler—and they were great friends. We all went to lunch; I think it was Kessler and Jim Krajeski. They all sat down together, but I was a little reluctant. Over lunch, my former analyst spoke up and told me, in essence, that he was glad that I had survived his treatment. He also said, "We're all entitled to mistakes and things are seen very differently today than they were fifteen or twenty years ago." It was really reassuring to me. Later, when I began speaking publicly about HIV, he invited me to give some lectures at Downstate Medical School in Brooklyn. I thought that was the complete turning of the screw—this guy who had tried to cure me was now calling on me to help. Life is funny.

JGLP: Are there any last things you want to say before we end?

DR. NICHOLS: Since I've come alive again in the last few months, I've really started to open up. I don't know how much time I've got left, but I really want to not just sit around and moan. I want to do things. I want to not focus on my limitations, but to focus on my abilities. To dare to perform, like doing this interview. I'm willing to fail, if that's what happens. If you don't try, you're guaranteed to fail. That's easy to say. I feel more like the old me.

People who have been important to me in my life—I've really made a point of getting back in touch with them. I've been occupying a lot of my time with that kind of effort now and it's very satisfying. Conversely, I've dropped people who really don't do anything for me. Who needs them?

I've almost died four times—don't wait for a fifth. Do it now. That's really good for me.

NOTES

1. See Joseph P. Merlino's interview with Bertram H. Schaffner, MD, Chapter 12 in this book.
2. Editor's Note: For details of those events, see Bayer, R. (1981), *Homosexuality and American Psychiatry: The Politics of Diagnosis.* New York: Basic Books.
3. Washington, DC, in 1971.
4. Dallas in 1972.
5. Editor's Note: See David Scasta's "John E. Fryer, MD, and the Dr. H. Anonymous Episode," Chapter 1 in this book.
6. Editor's Note: Hetrick and Martin were the founders of the Institute for the Protection of Lesbian and Gay Youth. After their deaths in the 1980s, it was renamed the Hetrick-Martin Institute.
7. Editor's Note: This was in 1978.
8. Editor's Note: In 1981, a multispecialty physicians' group was formed in New York City called New York Physicians for Human Rights. It disbanded for several years in the 1990s and later reformed as the New York Gay and Lesbian Physicians (NYGLP).
9. Dr. Bert Schaffner's apartment in New York has served as a meeting space for numerous groups over many years.
10. 1981, NYPHR.
11. Gay-related immune deficiency.
12. Gay Men's Health Crisis.

SELECTED BIBLIOGRAPHY

Nichols, S. E. & Reams, W. M. (1959), Serosal melanocytes in the PET mouse. *Virginia J. Science,* 10(4).

Nichols, S. E. & Reams, W. M. (1960), The occurrence and differentiation of melanocytes in the connective tissues of the PET mouse. *J. Emb. & Exp. Morph.,* 8(1):24-32.

Nichols, S. E. (1983), Psychiatric aspects of AIDS. *Psychosomatics,* 24(12):1083-1089.

Nichols, S. E. & Ostrow, D. G., eds. (1984), *Psychiatric Implications of Acquired Immune Deficiency Syndrome.* Washington, DC: American Psychiatric Press.

Nichols, S. E. (1985), Psychosocial reactions of persons with the acquired immunodeficiency syndrome. *Ann. Intern. Med.*, 103:765-767.

Nichols, S. E. (1986), Psychotherapy and AIDS. In: *Contemporary Perspectives on Psychotherapy with Lesbians and Gay Men*, ed. T. S. Stein, S. M. Woods & C. Cohen. New York: Plenum Press, pp. 209-239.

Chapter 11

Remembering Emery Hetrick, MD

Joyce Hunter

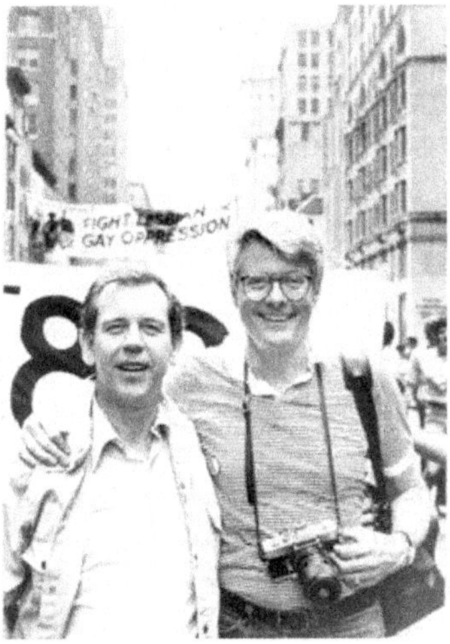

In November 1979, I was asked to speak before a New York political action group. This was a few weeks after the 1979 March on Washington for Lesbian and Gay Rights. Steve Ault and I had been co-coordinators of the march and we were asked to speak about the future of the lesbian and gay movement. It was at this meeting that I met Emery Hetrick, MD, a psychiatrist whom I had known by reputation from a featured photo-essay in *Life Magazine* ten years earlier.

Pioneer and Innovator

Emery Hetrick was born in Columbus, Ohio. He graduated from Ohio State University in 1953 and Cornell University College of Medicine in 1957. Emery served as a medical officer in the United States Navy. Emery had been the first psychiatrist hired by the Ackerman Family Institute, a pioneering organization in family therapy, where he trained under noted psychoanalyst and family therapist Nathan Ackerman. After starting the Mobile Crisis Unit at Gouverneur Hospital in downtown New York City (see the following paragraph), he also served as Chief of Psychiatric Emergency and Crisis Treatment Services at Harlem Hospital Center (1976-7199). When Emery died of AIDS at the age of fifty-six in

doi:10.1300/6049_12

1986, he was a highly respected Director of Medical Research for Pfizer Pharmaceuticals in New York.

In preparing to write about Emery and his work, I spoke with numerous colleagues and friends. They all remembered him as being, from the very beginning of his career, generous with his time and characterized by a willingness to take risks on behalf of people in need. One example of his early vision was his creation of the Mobile Crisis Unit at Gouverneur Hospital.[1] Emery was the first psychiatrist with the original mobile crisis team that included Lynn Hoffman, Kitty LePerrier, Carlos Martinez, and Lisa Schwab-Levy. Emery and his mental health team developed their plan for the Mobile Crisis Unit and implemented the program on East Broadway in New York City, an area outside the hospital's catchment area. In fact, the *Life Magazine* story I had read ten years before meeting Emery had featured both him and the Mobile Crisis Unit—a pioneering program, quite radical for its time. *Life* described it as taking psychiatry "off the couch and into the community."

Lisa Levy, who joined the Mobile Crisis Unit in the late 1960s, worked with Emery for eleven years. She recalls the team grew to include additional social workers, a nurse, three paraprofessionals, and a driver. The team worked together for several years. The program, funded through a $10 million grant from the National Institute of Health to Beth Israel Hospital, was designed to bring innovative mental health and psychiatric care to economically disadvantaged areas. The Mobile Crisis Unit was a bold experiment in community psychiatry; it intervened on behalf of individuals, often in crisis, referred by doctors, priests, welfare workers, and others in the community. The goal was to help these individuals without removing them from their community.

Emery, of course, had his critics. Among other things, he was called "an ambulance chaser." The critics predicted the program would not work. However, despite initial resistance, Emery's vision of community psychiatric care was eventually adopted, not only by many New York hospitals, but also by hospitals nationwide. The Mobile Crisis program was a success.

As a result of the 1969 *Life Magazine* article on the Mobile Crisis Unit, Emery received a request from a psychiatrist at a famous hospital in Zurich to come to New York and work with him for a week. She wanted to see how the program worked and if it was possible to adopt the model in Switzerland. This visit led to an official invitation to visit the Zurich hospital. Emery and some team members, including Lisa, traveled to Switzerland to assist the hospital staff in implementing the program there. As they stepped off the plane, the psychiatrist they had met in New York greeted them with a request: "I must ask you a great favor. We have our monthly psychiatrists' meeting tonight, and the doctor who was supposed to speak is not going to be there. Could Lisa [who speaks French and German] please fill in for him?" Emery responded, "Yes, of course, she can," without hesitation and without asking Lisa! He had confidence in her. That talk and the entire visit turned out well, with the Zurich hospital then adopting the Mobile Crisis Unit model. Today, there is a Mobile Crisis Unit in every hospital throughout Switzerland.

The Mobile Crisis team members I interviewed spoke of Emery's talent, his clinical mind and understanding of theory, his dedication to neglected populations, his tenderness, his uncanny ability to empathize with others, and how privileged they were to have known and worked with him. Emery spent several years at the Mobile Crisis Unit, before going on to become Director of Psychiatry at Gouverneur Hospital.

Compassionate Therapist

Emery was an analytical psychotherapist and also a superb family therapist. He could relate to all types of people. Rita Gazarik recalled Emery's gifts in working with families. One family they visited over a period of time included a mother and father, both survivors of the Holocaust, and their only daughter, a disturbed young woman who had become an Andy Warhol "groupie." She was involved with drugs that affected her brain functioning and caused her to become unpredictably psychotic. Emery was the first person in a long series of mental health professionals who could communicate with the daughter, who understood her psychotic language, and who gained the trust of the parents as well.

Rita still sees people who greet her and thank her for the work she and Emery did together. Recently, a former woman client told Rita how grateful she was when Emery helped her with her alcoholism. He took the woman to an Alcoholics Anonymous (AA) meeting, which she remembers as the beginning of her recovery process. It was really amazing, given his origins as a Midwest, small-town "WASP," how Emery emerged as sophisticated and brilliant in his field and a visionary in services needed for the LGBT community. People who have worked with him in various situations have also commented on Emery's interviewing skills, describing them as "classy," superb, and very professional, regardless of the circumstances. Emery taught his colleagues these skills.

Advocate

The Association of Gay and Lesbian Psychiatrists (AGLP) traces its roots to the late 1960s, when gay and lesbian members of the American Psychiatric Association (APA) met informally at the annual meetings.[2] In 1973, the APA removed homosexuality per se as a mental disorder from its diagnostic manual (DSM-II), facilitating a more open association of lesbian and gay psychiatrists. Eventually, a group called the Caucus of Homosexually Identified Psychiatrists (CHIP) was established in the mid-1970s. Later, this group would have representation in the APA Assembly and eventually change its name to the APA Caucus of Gay, Lesbian, and Bisexual Psychiatrists. The caucus members would also spin off a separate organization, but allied with the APA, the Association of Gay and Lesbian Psychiatrists. In response to a petition from CHIP in 1978, the APA also created a task force on gay and lesbian issues. This task force has since become a standing committee (Committee on Gay, Lesbian, and Bisexual Issues) that advises the APA on issues related to the mental health of GLB populations.

At the 1978 annual meeting of the American Psychiatric Association, a photo of Emery as an openly gay psychiatrist with his partner, Damien Martin, PhD, was displayed at a booth in the exhibition hall that featured the theme "Gay Love: Good Medicine." Emery loved doing it. Once he came out, all his energies went to addressing unmet issues within the gay community, and his skills and professionalism really helped the cause.

While gay and lesbian psychiatrists were organizing nationally in the late 1970s, they were also organizing locally. In the New York metropolitan area, this led to the creation of GLPNY (Gay and Lesbian Psychiatrists of New York)—and Emery was one of the people instrumental in that organization's creation and development. In the early years of GLPNY, Emery organized a consciousness-raising group, and I became involved with that group (GLPNY has always offered full membership to mental health professionals who are not psychiatrists). He had previously attended another consciousness-raising group and used that experience to serve as facilitator of the GLPNY group. Our group met for many months, and a number of people were a part of that group, many of whom are no longer with us. As a result of the work done in the consciousness-raising group, Emery, Gerry (E. Gerald) Dabbs, and Stuart Nichols,[3] helped form the first committee on gay, lesbian, and bisexual issues of the New York County District Branch of the APA.

Emery was also a co-founder and supporter of Senior Action in a Gay Environment (SAGE), a group providing social support and social services in New York. He could see that older gay people who lost lovers were mourning losses that they could not mourn in public, and that they needed support groups and help. Damien told me that Emery financially supported SAGE for a year, an example of his generosity with both his money and time when he thought an organization or an issue was important to the community. More than twenty years later, SAGE remains a thriving social support organization in New York City.

Institute for the Protection of Lesbian and Gay Youth

In 1979, Emery heard from a colleague working in a local hospital emergency room that a gay male teenager had been gang-raped at a homeless shelter, and that the boy, and not the rapists, was told that he would have to leave the shelter. Emery and Damien were determined to prevent this kind of treatment of gay youth from happening again.

That year, along with several others, Emery and Damien formed an education and advocacy group, the Institute for the Protection of Lesbian and Gay Youth (IPLGY)—which would eventually become the Hetrick-Martin Institute (HMI). I was a member of the founding group; when IPLGY incorporated, I became a member of the board, eventually serving as vice president. Although funding was a problem, both Emery and Damien felt we should move ahead with our plans. After many meetings at their apartment, IPLGY opened for services to lesbian, gay, bisexual, and transgender youth and their families in November 1983.

Early discussions had revolved around the issue of whether this agency would be educational and provide trainings or whether it would provide direct services to LGBT youth. Emery was influential in persuading the board that we could carry out both types of activities.

We felt that providing education for professionals and paraprofessionals who work with LGBT youth was essential. At that time, despite some social progress, many religious groups and people who had political influence continued to view homosexuality with fear and hatred. Still an issue today, society's negative attitudes toward homosexuality create special problems for LGBT youth, including shame and alienation, disruption of family ties, and isolation from peers. We knew there were many LGBT youth experiencing physical abuse, who were running away and who were homeless. Some were surviving through involvement in sex work. Unaware of any possible available social services—and often afraid of the consequences of disclosure—many young LGBT adolescents were discouraged from seeking the help they needed. While several youth agencies in the New York metropolitan area offered services to these youth at that time, only a few were equipped or wished to handle the specific problems of LGBT youth. Fear and lack of knowledge about homosexuality and transgender youth on the part of concerned agencies and their staff also added to the inadequacy of services.

At its inception, IPLGY was composed solely of the board of directors who carried out the organization's activities with the assistance of some volunteers. Early board members included Florence Vigilante, DSW, and Hattie Mitchell, PhD—both distinguished social workers; Marsha Day, Dr. Stephen Karakaskian, Paul Paroski, MD, a pediatrician, and Richard and Amy Ashworth, founders of the New York City Chapter of Parents and Friends of Lesbians and Gays (PFLAG).

We realized early on that the needs of LGBT youth and the dearth of services for and information about this population would necessitate an expansion of our services and activities. If we wanted to achieve our goals, it would require offering direct services, hiring a full-time professional staff, and finding the funds to hire that staff.

As a volunteer for the Student Health Society at Hunter College, I had developed an intake form, on a 3 × 5 card, for students, straight and gay, coming in for help to the Student Health Society office. This student-run health society kept students' personal health information confidential, collecting only the first name, the presenting problem, and any referral information. This service was an appealing alternative to the traditional counseling services available to students at the college, where records were kept of personal details of student interviews. Emery strongly urged me to obtain a social work degree. "You have all this data. You can write it up, but no one will listen. You need the credentials."

I enrolled in the Hunter School of Social Work in 1982, while still working with Emery and Damien in developing the new agency at the same time. It was a great time. I did my fieldwork at The Door and other agencies that serve adolescents, where I was able to get the kind of experience we would need at our new agency. By the time IPLGY opened in 1983, I was able, with Damien and Emery, to present a design of what the program should look like.

Some time after IPLGY began to offer services, Emery asked me to come to his apartment. He and Damien wanted me to meet a very special person who was aware of the institute's work. This donor, who wished to remain anonymous, after talking with Emery and Damien about the new agency, took $25,000 in cash out of his boot and placed it on their table. The next day he came back with another $25,000 in cash. With that $50,000, we were able to obtain a matching grant from the New York City Youth Bureau. Emery and Damien began to meet with the New York City Youth Bureau staff and New York State Division for Youth. We began to obtain the funding we needed to hire staff and obtain space for staff and professional volunteers to directly serve the young people. You could say the rest is history.

We first instituted a training and education program for professionals and paraprofessionals. We developed services, and we had carefully chosen professional volunteers. Initially, I was an unpaid staff member, eventually becoming qualified and hired as Director of Social Services and Clinical Supervisor. We hired additional social workers as we were able. I had had counseling training with supervision and had done counseling at Hunter College. After I graduated from social work school, I felt I would need to continue with clinical supervision. Emery was my clinical supervisor, and he was called in whenever we had someone who needed a psychiatric assessment. He also brought in Rita Gazarik, a social worker who had worked with him at the Mobile Crisis Unit, as a consultant to work with staff on family issues.

During that time, E. Gerald (Gerry) Dabbs, MD, was one of our consultants. Emery was not a child and adolescent specialist, so he sometimes asked colleagues to see youth who were having particular psychiatric problems. Dr. Dabbs would see these young people in his private office. Other child psychiatrists, including Richard Pleak, MD, and Dennis Anderson, MD, also helped with psychiatric evaluations and therapy—without charging fees.

Emery's long-term vision for the institute was to provide a mental health clinic with a family services component. He thought miles ahead but cautioned that the way to achieve that goal would be to go slowly, be patient, begin the programs, and then we would be able to obtain the documentation of need and the funding that we would need to move on to family services. This idea was very close to his heart. It has not happened, I think, at the scale he imagined. However, it is still happening.

Emery became ill in late 1984. It was a difficult time for everyone who cared about him, and for Damien especially. Even though Emery was ill and his health was deteriorating, he was still involved with the institute. He became ill shortly before the institute's Harvey Milk High School opened in 1985. In spite of his illness, he spoke and wrote eloquently about why this organization was needed, who these youth were, and what their needs were, responding to questions about them, primarily from other groups serving youth. He was able to give very clear explanations without pathologizing the youth. Some of the adolescents were disturbed, but most of them were very isolated and lonely and really needed to be part of a peer group and have adults who would be supportive and not criticize or exploit them. He was very proud that the institute was creating the first school for LGBT youth.

During this period, Emery and Damien wrote some really great articles together. A major paper, "Ego-Dystonic Homosexuality: A Developmental View" (1984), is still referred to in regard to development and clinical aspects of this population. Another important article written by them, "Designing an AIDS Risk Reduction Program for Gay Teenagers: Problems and Proposed Solutions," was published in 1987.

As the institute grew, I stepped down from the board of directors and became the Director of Social Services. IPLGY also began to develop a professional board, with individuals from business and funders who could help raise money, as well as service providers. Emery was very clear on not being totally dependent on government funds, as they can come and go given the political situation. He was very insightful about that.

Even when Emery was hospitalized, he continued to work on his vision for a family therapy program at the institute. Rita Gazarik remembers Emery dictating the research questions to address in pursuing funding for a family studies project. There is now a family program at the institute.

The institute's programs reflect the legacy of Emery, Damien, and those of us who worked with the agency early on: family and individual counseling, socialization program, drop-in center, with discussions, games, films, art, drama, outreach programs to high-risk youth, and the alternative high school program.

Friend and Mentor

I want to document Emery's and Damien's lives outside of their professional activities. People were able to see more of the professional side, and they often did not see the more personal side of them. They met each other at an AA meeting in the 1970s. Damien told me that when he saw Emery, he knew he would be spending the rest of his life with him.

During the time I worked with them, which was every weekend possible, they would take their car out of its garage, travel through the Lincoln Tunnel and make their way to the country, to their home in Accord, in the Hudson Valley. On weekends when Jan, my partner, and I would join them, we were in for a treat—many treats. Damien loved to cook and Emery loved gardening. I began taking pictures of Emery and Damien while there. Each weekend, after a full weekend of eating, gardening, and antiquing or touring, we would arrive back at their apartment late Sunday, have Damien's special soup, and we would begin, with Damien at the computer, to work on yet another grant application!

I will never forget the time that my mother was dying from cancer. Jan and I had spent the weekend with Emery and Damien at their house in the country, and on the way back I planned to stop and see my mother. Emery was very concerned about how I was feeling about her illness and the stress of trying to take care of her. He came with me to see her. He was so gentle and sensitive that he was able to get her to talk about how she was feeling. It meant so much to me, and she talked more about personal things in my subsequent visits with her.

What people may not know about Emery was that he was an art historian, and he loved going to museums. My minor in college was art, so to go through art museums with him was fascinating. And he loved it; he really loved it. It was a tradition for Emery to spend New Year's Eve with Gregory Bateson and Margaret Mead. It was also traditional for Emery and Damien to go with Jan, Rita, and me to the Metropolitan Museum on New Year's Day, then for tea at the Plaza. Our annual holiday visit to the museum was an anticipated event. As we moved through the museum, he loved to discuss everything about each selected painting—the painter, the period, the politics. You had to be patient, though!

On many occasions I went with Emery to the opera. He took me to my first opera, so I will never forget that. While Damien was not as enthusiastic about the opera, he was, however, an actor, and a good one.

It was fascinating to hear the two of them discuss an issue. They had many intellectual debates, sometimes heated, often one talking and the other writing. This could go on for days. They would argue, but their arguments were very constructive. Jan and I would just listen in amazement. They were very affectionate, but they also really liked to discuss and debate issues. Sometimes their debates were heated. But their love for each other was unwavering. I know that their discussions were one of the things Damien missed most after Emery died.

As they approached the end of their lives, the institute became the focus for them; they realized time was running out for them. Even with all he was dealing with, Emery made himself available to me and others when he could. For example, if Damien and I disagreed on a policy or activity, I would go to Emery and say, "I proposed this idea to Damien regarding programming, and Damien said he didn't think it would work." I would give my explanation to Emery, and then the two of them would discuss it that night. The next day Damien would say, "Well, Emery and I talked about it, and we decided that your idea is not bad. Let's try it." Both were real mentors for me; I had fathers and brothers all in one. That is how I felt about them. They were very generous.

HIV/AIDS

Emery and I also served on then Governor Cuomo's New York State Lesbian and Gay Task Force. It was a good thing because, in 1981, AIDS came into the picture, and Emery saw that we needed to start early with adolescents. We began advocating for needed prevention programs for adolescents, particularly given the long incubation period and lack of early symptoms for HIV. We needed to do something immediately. We developed a comic book series, *Tales of the Closet,* about HIV prevention and stigma for and about kids with Ivan Velez, a young artist. This series was the first of its kind. Then we developed an intervention program. It was fulfilling to be able to do this work.

Then we, Damien, Emery, and I, founded the AIDS and Adolescents Network for New York City. But Emery was becoming symptomatic, more frequently feeling ill, at that time. Emery's illness affected us all and made all of us determined to establish the agency as a stable and credible institution.

I remember Emery and Damien bought me a suit in recognition of my representing the Coalition for Lesbian and Gay Rights at the City Hall hearings on the gay rights bill that passed that year—after many years of lobbying. Emery said, "Joyce, you are going to wear a suit or a skirt when you go out to represent the agency at government meetings." I remember coming back to the institute one day after a presentation at a governmental meeting, and the kids noticed me in a skirt. They said, "Joyce has legs!" I reported to Emery and Damien, "See what I did for you guys. I got dressed in drag." They taught me how important it was that people be able to hear what you are saying, and that you are not what you are or are not wearing. I learned about professionalism from them, and to make sure you understand your own biases. I heard Emery once say that communities are based on the institutions you have built. That is what makes a community, the institutions that you provide for your people.

Emery himself would always be dressed in a three-piece suit with a white shirt, with his Phi Beta Kappa key. He would dress like that, whether he was interviewing a youth in a stairwell or if he was talking with a psychotic patient in the patient's home. I remember a very hot day one summer, when we were walking up his block and bumped into a neighbor. The neighbor asked him why he was wearing a shirt and a tie with the shirt all the way buttoned. He said, "Because I'm an Anglo-Saxon Protestant. I'm a WASP, and that's how I'm supposed to dress."

Eventually Damien became Executive Director of IPLGY, adding to his responsibilities as a professor at NYU and caring for Emery. Taking on this role was part of forwarding their vision, but it did put more stress on him. Emery stayed involved all through his illness, doing what he could and visiting the office when he could. I remember one time, a lot of these young people did not believe that you can grow old and be gay, be gay and grow old, so he sat in a group, he and Damien, did some group work with a group of boys, and talked about how they met and that you can stay in relations, and you can have a good life.

Harvey Milk High School

In the year prior to the opening of the Harvey Milk High School, we saw many young people hanging out at the institute during school hours. Young people could come into the institute before 3 p.m. if they had an appointment with a counselor or if they were out of school early to be mentored or tutored. However, hanging out during school hours was not allowed. After talking to those youth who were not there for appointments with staff, we found most of them had been victimized at their schools. Many of them had been verbally harassed or threatened; some had been physically attacked or beaten, making school an unsafe place for them. In many cases, the teachers and school staff had turned the other way when these incidents occurred. Unsurprisingly, this kind of school climate undermined the ability of these students to obtain an education, leading many of them to drop out of school.

It was then that Steve Ashkinazy, MSW, another institute social worker, and I decided that these youth were entitled to an education and that they needed an alternative school. We co-founded the Harvey

Milk High School. The school opened on April 15, 1985, in a church building in the Village. The school is still part of the New York City Board of Education's alternative high school program.

On opening day, there was a lot of media craziness. Except for the threats, one would think we were famous. We posted guards at the doors to the school in response to these threats. Photographers were taking pictures as the kids were trying to run away from them; they were stalking the students. Fortunately, some good things came from the notoriety. There was a front-page *New York Times* article and a very positive editorial. And the story traveled around the world. People were calling me from Spain and Japan. Others with negative things to say were referred to Damien. Damien had very good knowledge of the Bible. If anybody wanted to talk about "what the Bible says," we sent that person to Damien. Emery spoke often and eloquently to the media and others who questioned the work of the institute and the school. He was able to discuss clinical and policy issues in a way to which people responded well. He knew how to talk with people who were very negative about homosexuality and the lesbian and gay community. His caring showed through.

In June 1985, in spite of being ill, Emery marched in the Lesbian and Gay Pride Parade, proudly holding a Harvey Milk High School banner.

During that period, Emery became increasingly frustrated and angry, as he realized he would not be alive to attend to the institute's work and to see his other visions come to fruition. Emery died in 1986, but his work lives on.

Writing this profile of Emery Hetrick has brought back many fond memories—the joy of working with him, and with Damien, and the honor of being able to share in bringing to fruition their vision of an organization serving LGBT youth. These two men left behind a brilliant legacy. There are very few people who have had the luxury of having Emery as their mentor, teacher, and close friend. I was one of the lucky ones to be part of Emery's and Damien's legacies.

NOTES

1. Rita Gazarik, Lee Grove, and Lisa Schwab-Levy (group interview June 2004).

2. The group members referred to themselves as the Gay-P-A. See Bayer, R. (1981), *Homosexuality and American Psychiatry: The Politics of Diagnosis.* New

York: Basic Books; Kenn Ashley's interview with Stuart E. Nichols, MD, Chapter 10 in this book; and David Scasta's article on John E. Fryer, MD, and the Dr. H. Anonymous episode, Chapter 1 in this book.

3. See Kenn Ashley's interview with Stuart E. Nichols, MD, Chapter 10 in this book.

REFERENCES

Hetrick, E.S. & Martin, A.D. (1984), Ego-dystonic homosexuality: A developmental view. In: *Innovations in Psychotherapy with Homosexuals,* ed. E.S. Hetrick & T.S. Stein. Washington DC: American Psychiatric Association Press, pp. 2-21.

Martin, A.D. & Hetrick, E.S. (1987), Designing an AIDS risk reduction program for gay teenagers: Problems and proposed solutions. In: *Biobehavioral Control of AIDS,* ed. D.G. Ostrow. New York: Irvington, pp. 137-152.

SECTION III: GAY AND LESBIAN PSYCHIATRISTS OF NOTE

Chapter 12

An Interview with Bertram H. Schaffner, MD

Joseph P. Merlino

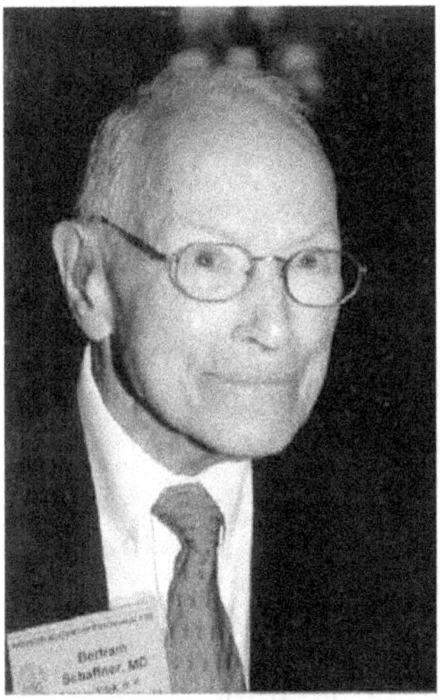

The editors of the *Journal of Gay & Lesbian Psychotherapy* believe it is very important to profile the leaders within psychiatry and psychotherapy who have had a major impact on the work of gay and lesbian therapists and also gay and lesbian patients. We have assembled an initial group who, in our judgment, have made signal achievements in this area.

Dr. Bertram H. Schaffner was the editors' unanimous first choice to initiate this occasional series. Dr. Schaffner was born in Erie, Pennsylvania, on November 12, 1912. His parents were of German-Jewish descent and Bert, as most of us know him, lived in a mostly German community. Bert visited his grandparents in Germany several times as a child and attended a German public school, more autocratic than permissive, where he was forced to write with his right hand although he was left-handed.

Bert skipped grades regularly and entered Harvard University at age fifteen where he received superior grades. He later transferred to

This chapter appeared originally under the same title in *Journal of Gay & Lesbian Psychotherapy* 5(1):85-99. Copyright 2001 The Haworth Press, Inc.

American Psychiatry and Homosexuality: An Oral History
Published by The Haworth Press, Inc., 2007. All rights reserved.
doi:10.1300/6049_13

the Honors Program at Swarthmore College and majored in English literature and philosophy. He received his medical degree from Johns Hopkins Medical School in 1937. Residency training in neurology, neurosurgery, and neuropathology followed at New York's Mount Sinai Hospital. Dr. Schaffner's psychiatric training was completed at Bellevue Hospital and at the New York State Psychiatric Institute.

He was called to active duty in the army upon completion of his residency in April 1941, eight months before Pearl Harbor. Dr. Schaffner was assigned to do psychiatric assessments of draftees for the Selective Service System. In this role, he was to determine if these draftees were mentally fit to serve in the army and to weed out people likely to break down under stress, or people who might "undermine morale" among the troops. It was clear to Dr. Schaffner that the army wanted homosexuals to be identified and excluded from military service. Here he demonstrated his wonderful ability to help people through difficulty while doing everything possible to maintain their dignity, self-respect, and safety. Those who were homosexual and believed they could not serve were assisted out of the army by Dr. Schaffner for other reasons. This way they could retain their civilian lives with no one knowing of their homosexuality. Those gay men who wished to serve were allowed to do so with a warning from Dr. Schaffner about what awaited them in the military. In August 1944, he was sent to Camp Gordon, Georgia, to prepare to go overseas with the 10th Armored Division as the division neuropsychiatrist, where he saw active combat during the Battle of the Bulge.

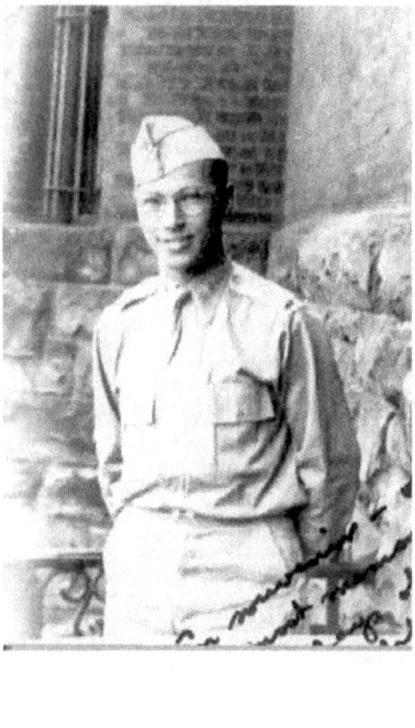

Before the war ended, he was sent for a month's training in neurology to London's Queen's Square Hospital. This proved useful in his next assignment at the Nuremberg trails at the end of 1945, where he was to keep alive Kaltenbrunner, a high-level Nazi war criminal, after he had suffered a life-threatening subarachnoid hemorrhage. Kaltenbrunner survived, underwent the trial for war crimes, and was executed.

At the end of World War II, at the suggestion of Margaret Mead, he was invited to stay on in military service to work on the denazification process in occupied Germany by the American Military Government. He was designated Chief of the Information Control Division's Screening Center. As a result of this assignment, he wrote the book *Fatherland: A Study of Authoritarianism in the German Family,* which was published in 1948 with prefaces by Margaret Mead and child psychiatrist Dr. David M. Levy.

From 1949 till 1953, Dr. Schaffner underwent psychoanalytic training at the William Alanson White Institute, with Clara Thompson as his analyst.[1] He also studied under Frieda Fromm-Reichmann, Ralph Crowley, and Erich Fromm. In 1958 he was elected president of the William Alanson White Psychoanalytic Society. At the White Institute, he has taught and supervised candidates in psychoanalysis up to the present time.

From 1948 to 1960, he served on the Expert Committee for Mental Health of the United Nations. During that time, he was a member of the Committee on International Relations at the Group for the Advancement of Psychiatry, and he chaired that committee until 1980.

From 1948 to 1962, while principally in private practice in New York City, he brought together various groups from West Indian islands, to form the U.S. Caribbean Aid to Mental Health, of which he was executive director and fund-raiser for many years. This organization stimulated mental health associations in the Caribbean Islands, promoted change in Island government programs for the care of the mentally ill, sent U.S. volunteers to serve in their hospitals and prisons, and worked to reduce the stigma of mental illness. This ultimately led to the donation of funds and establishment of a Department of Psychiatry in the University of the West Indies in Jamaica.

His career continues to be a rich and remarkable one. From the onset of the AIDS epidemic, Dr. Schaffner has been on the front lines caring for patients and caregivers. He was instrumental in providing group psychotherapy for physicians with AIDS, along with his colleague Dr. Stuart Nichols,[2] from 1985 until the present time.

Dr. Schaffner has conducted his private practice for over forty-six years, travels extensively throughout the world, has collected art primarily from Asia, is a supporter of the Asian Art Department of the Brooklyn Museum of Art, and is a member of the Museum's Acquisition Committee.

Dr. Schaffner has produced numerous publications to date on topics from "AIDS" to "working abroad" and has more in the works. His latest paper, soon to be published, is titled "Androgyny in Indian Culture and Art: Psychoanalytic Implications."[3] He has also completed a genealogical history of his family which was published upon his eightieth birthday.

He is a Live Fellow of the American Medical Association, the American Psychiatric Association, and the American Academy of Psychoanalysis. Dr. Schaffner has been a member of the Group for the Advancement of Psychiatry (GAP) since 1950, and was the founding chairperson of GAP's newest committee, the Committee on Human Sexuality. In 2000, the Analytic Press published his committee's monograph on antihomosexual bias within psychiatry. Astonishingly, with a life full of achievements as just outlined, Dr. Schaffner remains a low-key and modest individual. Indeed, one may "know" him for many years and still be amazed to learn how much more there is to learn about his remarkably multifaceted man.

The *Journal of Gay & Lesbian Psychotherapy* interviewed Dr. Schaffner in the fall of 1999. Since he has witnessed and experienced so much in his rich life, this interview could have been on just about any topic one can imagine. On the eave of the publication of the GAP committee's monograph, *Homosexuality and the Mental Health Professions: The Impact of Bias,* he discusses how the difficulties and pains experienced from homophobia (his personal, society's, and psychiatry's) have influenced his interest in Indian art, and how Indian art may have helped him to heal.

JGLP: I know that one of the things that you are passionate about is your love and interest in Indian art. How long have you been involved in studying and collecting Indian art?

DR. SCHAFFNER: Actually, since about 1967—thirty-two years.

JGLP: Can you tell us how that became such an interest of yours, and how it relates to your work as a psychotherapist and analyst?

DR. SCHAFFNER: Well, actually, when I went to India, I was fleeing the psychological and organizational work that I had been doing in the Caribbean. I really did not travel to India for "professional" reasons. I stayed away from psychological meetings. I did not go to meet other psychiatrists. I had just finished a very painful period—the painful ending of my time in the Caribbean where I had concentrated on establishing mental health associations and programs on nearly all the islands. At that time, you see, it was a period of political crisis concerning black and white relations—civil rights. And I had to terminate my work in the Caribbean because it was difficult for West Indians to accept a white executive director when they were struggling for power and the right to have more control over their own lives. Blacks had to assert their own leadership. I knew this, and I accepted it. However, I suffered intensely over the fact that my homosexuality was used as the excuse to justify my removal. This hostile act of unnecessary public embarrassment hurt me very deeply. I am sure that this played a large part in the depression that I went through for nearly two years after leaving the Caribbean, to which I had devoted so much of myself and my emotions. In India, I purposely stayed away from everything organizational, academic, and professional—everything political. The trip to India assisted in my personal recovery.

Going to India at that time also happened to coincide with a period in my personal analysis when I was feeling somewhat disillusioned with the field of psychoanalysis. In retrospect, I was probably getting over the original utopian premises in early psychoanalytical thinking! I am sure that I was also very disappointed in the psychoanalytic establishment's attitudes toward homosexuality. At the White Institute, Clara Thompson had died, and the new atmosphere was not hospitable toward homosexual issues. My trip to India also happened to be under the auspices of the Brooklyn Museum of Art, a serious study workshop on Indian art and culture, with a superb international faculty. I immersed myself in my first contact with Asian peoples, which had the unexpected advantage of taking place in an English-speaking country, where I could communicate easily. Another unexpected benefit was that it helped me deal with my own internal homophobia, which, I think, actually helped to prepare me to participate in the newly formed GLB Caucus at the American Psychiatric Association, around 1978 to 1980, where I met other openly gay psychiatrists.

JGLP: This was your first period of really coming in contact with openly gay physicians?

DR. SCHAFFNER: Yes. Because prior to that time, gay doctors were often afraid to have other doctors, gay or straight, know that they were gay. We were so afraid of anyone revealing our homosexuality. We did not know whether to trust others, even gay doctors. At that time, it was vitally important to keep everything secret, since physicians could lose their licenses for what was then known as "moral turpitude."

JGLP: So how did your experience with Indian culture help you to explore your sexuality?

DR. SCHAFFNER: In the India period, I dealt with issues like my own prudishness. Indian art was the first I encountered that was openly and comfortably sexual, not "covered up," as in much of Western, especially Victorian, art. No fig leaves. Big, nurturing, abnormally full and rounded, voluptuous breasts. The lingam (penis) being the public, central symbol of God in the Hindu religion, the first object seen when entering a Hindu temple. Indian art delights in depicting sexual attraction and caressing, affectionate love and even displays sexual acts formerly described as "perverted" in temple murals.

Although I also learned that present-day Indians (thanks to 300 years of British colonization) are trained not to express sexual attraction and affection in public, for example, hugging or kissing in public, they have not come to feel (compared to the West) that sexuality is "dirty," "shameful," or "bad." The Hindu religion emphasizes the delightful, divine, irresistible, almost magical pull of sexuality, not to mention its all-important connection with reproduction and parenthood, the ultimate goal of life. However, sexual feelings are regarded as essentially private, not for public behavior. All of this was very helpful to me in dispelling my own prudishness, and I began to travel to India frequently.

As for homosexuality, it is strictly frowned upon in India. It is absolutely essential to be married and to produce children. Human life was not considered fulfilled without having produced a child. Yet, there are many homosexuals in India: many of them are married and feel it vital to keep it secret. Some have divorced and emigrated to foreign countries, at great financial and emotional cost. Sometimes a man's married state may give him sufficient protection that he may be free to pursue his true interests. Nevertheless, I found many Indians who were comfortable with their homosexuality, despite the severe social disapproval, and who helped me to be comfortable as well, considerably different from my general experience at home.

Then there was also the whole matter of androgyny, which had been a major problem for me. In India you feel that the men are strong; at the same time you feel they are gentle and that their gentleness is acceptable, in fact culturally desirable. I felt very much at home with their gentleness. It also began to make me feel more comfortable with my own "sissyness," which I had always been at such pains to conceal. To be soft, tender, gentle is not a negative quality among Indians.

JGLP: As you talk about it, one can really hear the healing quality that your journey to India had on you.

DR. SCHAFFNER: It was almost life-saving in some ways.

JGLP: In terms of making you whole?

DR. SCHAFFNER: Yes.

JGLP: One can see the parallels between the Indian not showing affection and love publicly while being very intimate and expressive in private and what gay life has been for so many years.

DR. SCHAFFNER: Right. A very good point. I would say my life in America had always made me feel unwanted, and that I must not talk about my real feelings and life. Indians have a way of being very curious about your life. They would not ask directly about homosexuality, but they usually become quite concerned about how a person manages to live alone, without a wife. They assume that one must always have someone in his life, each taking care of the other. A premium is put upon interdependence and closeness. No emphasis on "rugged individualism"! The Indian view of American analysis is that we train people to aloneness, which they feel is pathological—to need other people is a sign of health. They see successful interpersonal relations as a healthy goal in living, not the historical goal in Freudian theory, achieving successful heterosexuality, which they seem to take for granted as everyone's natural ability. Perhaps this may account for the fact that I have not infrequently found Indians able to accept a successful male bonding within the family, more easily than in many Western fundamentalist families.

JGLP: One of the things that has always impressed me about you is how you have this very understated way of bringing people together. It appears that relationships and friendships evolve from the different groups that meet in your home or that you bring together. I always wondered how you made it seem so easy to do that. It very much resonates with what you are talking about in terms of India—that people should not be alone; people should come together. Were you like that most of your life?

DR. SCHAFFNER: I must have been. I felt so lonely as a child, an outcast, because I was frequently "found out" for being interested in sex with other kids. Families would often tell me that I could never come back! I developed a pattern of giving parties at my home, probably as a way of keeping contact with people. Maybe I was afraid to see people alone. It seemed safer if I saw them at a party I was hosting.

This doesn't mean that I felt less lonely. I always longed to feel acceptable but despaired that could ever be. I remained intensely interested in other people and tried to understand them. Perhaps because I felt unwanted, I made it a point not to reject anyone. I cultivated tolerance. I always felt that I was going out toward people. It is interesting that you say I do this in a quiet way.

I have a lot of very naïve assumptions. I assume that people will like each other! Not necessarily very realistic. But I think I have been optimistic that people will find interest in each other, perhaps because I do.

JGLP: It sounds like you've always been that way.

DR. SCHAFFNER: Funny, isn't it? Maybe because I felt so unwanted in Erie, Pennsylvania, but my life was not wholly confined to Erie. Every other year I went to Europe to visit my grandparents. I usually found people there much more accepting of me, much kinder. I always felt relieved when I went abroad. Maybe that was the beginning of my interest in cross-cultural psychiatry, trying to understand and bridge the two kinds of cultures that I lived in alternately.

JGLP: You went to Europe every other year for the summer?

DR. SCHAFFNER: For a couple of months, yes. Three times I went with my family for six months. The other times it was for shorter visits, until my grandparents died.

JGLP: How did that work out with your schooling?

DR. SCHAFFNER: It was not easy. On the longer visits, I attended German schools.

JGLP: What was that like?

DR. SCHAFFNER: I was used to the freedom of American schools, and, of course, I had to learn German. Also, I was left-handed, which was unacceptable in Germany. I was forced to write with the right hand, which I found embarrassingly awkward. And I didn't like being slapped on the hand with a ruler for making mistakes.

Interestingly enough, having been ostracized at home for sexual activities with other children, I was surprised to find that my little German cousins, with whom I was always put in the same bedroom, seemed to be just as interested in sexual play as myself, but there was no aura of "badness" or punishment, much to my surprise and relief.

JGLP: Was that during young adolescence?

DR. SCHAFFNER: Ages seven, ten, and twelve.

JGLP: So you really had a broad exposure that many of us don't have in terms of living in two countries?

DR. SCHAFFNER: Yes, different cultures. And I felt less fear of being unwanted in other countries. I think this contributed to my yearning to live a more openly gay life and harboring resentment that in my own country I had to hide what I felt to be so innate, so natural. I think you are helping me to bring out a strong underlying unconscious motivation in my life.

JGLP: I know, too, that you have had a hand in founding numerous gay committees and organizations. Do you see that same dynamic operating in that?

DR. SCHAFFNER: Yes. For me, it may have been easier to reach out to a group than to an individual. Perhaps that was my way of asking for help—to bring things together.

JGLP: But in that very process, you are bringing a number of people who may not have known each other together, and again that quiet way of uniting people for a common good seems to be operating.

DR. SCHAFFNER: As you know, Stu Nichols, to whom I always want to give a lot of credit, was the brave person who started the Gay Psychiatrists of New York (GPNY).[4] He, Emery Hetrick, and Damien Martin[5] were the sparkers of ideas who got things going and then invited me in to develop the project. It was perfect for me. Once the idea took root, one of my contributions was to write letters, to try to build the much needed community of gay psychiatrists and other mental health workers. I used to write them frequently, sharing the news of gay liberation efforts.

JGLP: That was with GPNY?

DR. SCHAFFNER: Yes. Stu Nichols and I also were involved very early with the AIDS epidemic, he through his connection with the Addiction Service at Beth Israel Hospital, and I when I was called upon to treat a hypomanic AIDS patient at New York Hospital. Because of the hysteria over HIV infection, Stu and I developed methods to help AIDS patients without their condition being revealed. He started a low-cost clinic at Beth Israel, where he treated the women's group and I the men. Together we also conducted a "secret" and totally confidential support group for HIV-positive physicians. This group has continued to the present day.

JGLP: You also have had a hand in starting other things as well. For example, the Committee on Human Sexuality within the Group for the Advancement of Psychiatry (GAP).

DR. SCHAFFNER: Yes. That was very much mine. That was really my initiative.

JGLP: I am aware that many gay professional groups regularly meet at your home in New York City. Your home has always been sort of a "Grand Central Station" for the gay mental health community!

DR. SCHAFFNER: It began in the 1950s. I had used my home as a meeting place for the new Caribbean Federation for Mental Health. That was an all-black group. It was not common then for a white person in a white neighborhood to invite eighty blacks into his home. Yet, it was something I felt it was important to do. And it worked out well for many years.

JGLP: So you were not apprehensive when it came time to host gay meetings?

DR. SCHAFFNER: No. It was not the first time in my life. In my childhood, my parents had been very progressive and had the courage to associate with so-called "leftist groups." When Marion Anderson came to Erie to sing, my parents invited her to stay in our house, as no hotel would take a black guest at that time! I was president of a "Liberal Club" while I was in college. So I guess I was used to sticking my neck out to demonstrate what I stood for, and, of course, there was a great reward in associating with interesting, new people. You could say that I followed a family tradition of being on the side of the underdog. However, when I became the underdog, that kind of support was not given to me. When my father learned that I was gay, I had to threaten suicide in order to be allowed to go on with my college education. This is all part of my trying to respond to your question about my seeming to be at ease with people.

JGLP: You've talked to a number of people and given many interviews. I wonder if there was an area or topic within those interviews that was not asked, that you felt was really important to put out there about you, about your life and your work—something unknown about you that you would like people to know about you.

DR. SCHAFFNER: It's a marvelous question. I have felt that there was something very central about me that I have never talked about to anybody, and I don't know quite what it is. But, I think . . . I guess I'm approaching it in reverse, but it's the best I can do. I'm really very romantic. And I think I wanted more than anything else to have a lover for all my life. And it's so easy to blame other people as if it's their fault. But, in trying to think what has made it not work out for me, I've been trying to look at the things in my own life that worked against it. I think a part of it was what is called internalized homophobia—feeling that if I expressed myself and joined my life with somebody else, I would become completely ostracized. Part of that was substantiated by the treatment I received in high school and my fears about my career as a doctor. It was legally dangerous when I became a doctor in 1937. I could have lost my license immediately for being gay. Today, I don't think anyone believes that a doctor would lose his license for being homosexual. I would certainly have been kicked out of medical school, and the same with the army. I had many fears that having a relationship would reveal to everyone that I was homosexual, and that it would reflect badly on me socially and professionally.

I was too idealistic about human relations when I was younger. I really did not understand the difference between sex and love. Until very late in life, I did not comprehend how people could be in love with one person and still be sexually attracted to someone else. No doubt I was also afraid to be involved. Nevertheless, I have had three or four important loving relationships. I feel I am much more understanding now, and I feel very much at peace about it. I believe that I have forgiven myself for these mistakes.

I hope that the people I loved have also found a way to forgive me. Maturing in this area of life, I believe, has probably made me more effective as a therapist. I wish I had known at age forty-eight what I now know at eighty-eight! But I do have the good fortune to be much cared about, and I share deeply in the happiness of others.

NOTES

1. Editor's Note: Dr. Schaffner's account of his personal analysis with Clara Thompson, the White Institute's first director, can be found in the interview by Steven Goldman (1995), The difficulty of being a gay psychoanalyst during the last fifty years: An interview with Dr. Bertram Schaffner. In: *Disorienting Sexualities,* ed. T. Domenici & R. Lesser. New York: Routledge, pp. 243-254.

2. Editor's Note: Stuart Nichols, MD, is a past president of AGLP who, until he was disabled by illness several years ago, was a significant advocate for gay and lesbian issues in the American Psychiatric Association. Dr. Nichols' interview is included as Chapter 10 of this book.

3. Editor's Note: See Schaffner, B. (2001), Androgyny in Indian culture and art: Psychoanalytic implications. *J. American Academy Psychoanalysis,* 29:113-125.

4. Editor's Note: Now Gay and Lesbian Psychiatrists of New York (GLPNY).

5. Editor's Note: The late Damien Martin, PhD, and his life partner, the late Emery Hetrick, MD, were co-founders of the Harvey Milk School and its parent organization, the Institute for the Protection of Gay and Lesbian Youth, which posthumously came to bear their names as the Hetrick-Martin Institute.

SELECTED BIBLIOGRAPHY

Books and Monographs

Schaffner, B. (1948), *Fatherland: A Study of Authoritarianism in the German Family.* New York: Columbia University Press.

Schaffner, B., ed. (1950), *Health and Human Relations in Germany: Report of the Second Conference on Problems of Health and Human Relations in Germany,* December 10-15, 1950, Williamsburg, VA. New York: Josiah Macy Jr. Foundation.

Schaffner, B., ed. (1954), *Group Processes: Transactions of the First Conference.* New York: Josiah Macy Jr. Foundation.

Schaffner, B., ed. (1955), *Group Processes: Transactions of the Second Conference.* New York: Josiah Macy Jr. Foundation.

Schaffner, B., ed. (1956), *Group Processes: Transactions of the Third Conference.* New York: Josiah Macy Jr. Foundation.

Schaffner, B., ed. (1957), *Group Processes: Transactions of the Fourth Conference.* New York: Josiah Macy Jr. Foundation.

Schaffner, B., ed. (1958), *Group Processes: Transactions of the Fifth Conference.* New York: Josiah Macy Jr. Foundation.

Group for the Advancement of Psychiatry (2000), *Homosexuality and the Mental Health Professions: The Impact of Bias.* Committee on Human Sexuality, B. Schaffner, Chair. Hillsdale, NJ: The Analytic Press.

Articles

Hohman, L.B. & Schaffner, B. (1947), Sex lives of unmarried men. *Amer. J. of Sociol.,* 7(6):501-507.

Schaffner, B. (1949), Book review of *Doctors of Infamy. Saturday Review of Literature,* March 12.

MacGregor, F.C. & Schaffner, B. (1950), Screening patients for nasal-plastic operations: A psychological study. *Psychosom. Med.,* 12(5):277-291.

Schaffner, B. (1955), Animal studies and human behavior. *Human Organization,* 15(1).

Schaffner, B. (1959), The individual, the family and the boss. In: *Emotional Forces in the Family,* ed. S. Liebman. New York: J.B. Lippincott Co.

Schaffner, B. (1959), Thoughts about therapy today. *Mental Hygiene,* 43(3), July.

Schaffner, B. (1963), Aims and results of the Curacao Conference. In: *Family Relationships: Proceedings of the Fourth Caribbean Conference for Mental Health,* April 16-23.

Schaffner, B. (1963), Special problems in setting up a mental health program in an international region: The Caribbean. *World Mental Health,* 15(2).

Schaffner, B. (1972), The cultural background. In: "Devi" and Transcultural Psychiatry, round table discussion, Transcultural Psychiatry Workshop, American Academy of Psychoanalysis. *J. of Contemp. Psychoanal.,* 8(2):190-193.

Schaffner, B. (1977), Contrasts and similarities in the handling of emotions in two different cultures. *Hiroshima Forum for Psychology,* 4:59-67.

Schaffner, B. (1985), Emotional reactions of medical personnel and intimates of persons with AIDS. *Forum of American Academy of Psychoanalysis,* 29(2): 10-13.

Schaffner, B. (1986), Psychological impact of AIDS upon the social environment, health care providers, families and friends and methods of modification. In *Proceedings of the Second International Conference on AIDS,* Paris, 1986, pp. 295-298.

Schaffner, B. (1986), Reactions of medical personnel and intimates to persons with AIDS. In: *Psychotherapy and the Memorable Patient,* ed. M. Stern. Binghamton, NY: The Haworth Press, pp. 67-80. Reprinted in: *Behavioral Aspects of AIDS,* ed. D.G. Ostrow. New York: Plenum Medical Books, 1990, pp. 341-354.

Schaffner, B. (1987), Review of *The AIDS Movie. Hosp. and Comm. Psychiat.,* 38(6):567-568.

Schaffner, B. (1987), Some thoughts about AIDS. *J. Subst. Abuse,* 4(3-4):141-142.

Defries, Z. & Schaffner, B. (1988), Media fever. *Newsletter of the New York County District Branch, American Psychiatric Association,* 11(3):2-13.

Schaffner, B. (1989), Ask the board: Case II discussion from psychiatry. *J. Gay & Lesb. Psychother.,* 1(2):9-12.

Schaffner, B. (1990), Psychotherapy with HIV-infected persons. *New Directions for Mental Health Services,* 48:5-20.

Schaffner, B. (1994), The crucial and difficult role of the psychotherapist in the treatment of the HIV-positive patient. *J. Amer. Acad. Psychoanal.,* 22(3):505-518.

Schaffner, B. (1996), Modifying psychoanalytic methods when treating HIV-positive patients. *J. Amer. Acad. Psychoanal.,* 25(1):123-141. Reprinted in: *Hope and Mortality: Psychodynamic Approaches to AIDS and HIV,* ed. M. Blechner. Hillsdale, NJ: The Analytic Press, 1997, pp. 63-79.

Chapter 13

An Interview with Martha J. Kirkpatrick, MD

Vernon A. Rosario

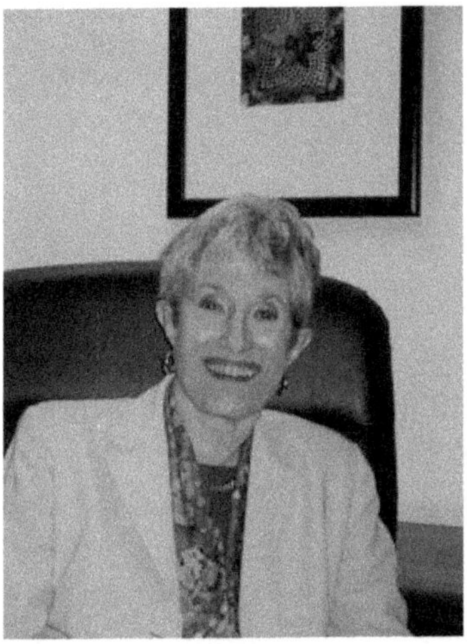

Martha J. Kirkpatrick has been a longtime leader in psychiatry and psychoanalysis, both as a woman and an "out" lesbian. Practicing psychiatry for over fifty years, she continues to revel in the psychoanalytic treatment of patients. As a dedicated, challenging, and much sought-after supervisor, Dr. Kirkpatrick has mentored numerous psychoanalysts and psychiatrists in Los Angeles. She has particularly been a mentor to a long line of gay psychiatry residents, including this interviewer. She has published extensively on the psychodynamics of female sexuality, psychotherapy with lesbians, and lesbian parenting. She is also a member of the editorial board of the *Journal of Gay & Lesbian Psychotherapy*.

Martha Kirkpatrick was interviewed on a gorgeous Sunday afternoon at the lovely home, high in the Brentwood hills, that she shares

This chapter appeared originally under the same title in *Journal of Gay & Lesbian Psychotherapy* 6(1):87-98. Copyright 2002 The Haworth Press, Inc.

American Psychiatry and Homosexuality: An Oral History
Published by The Haworth Press, Inc., 2007.
doi:10.1300/6049_14

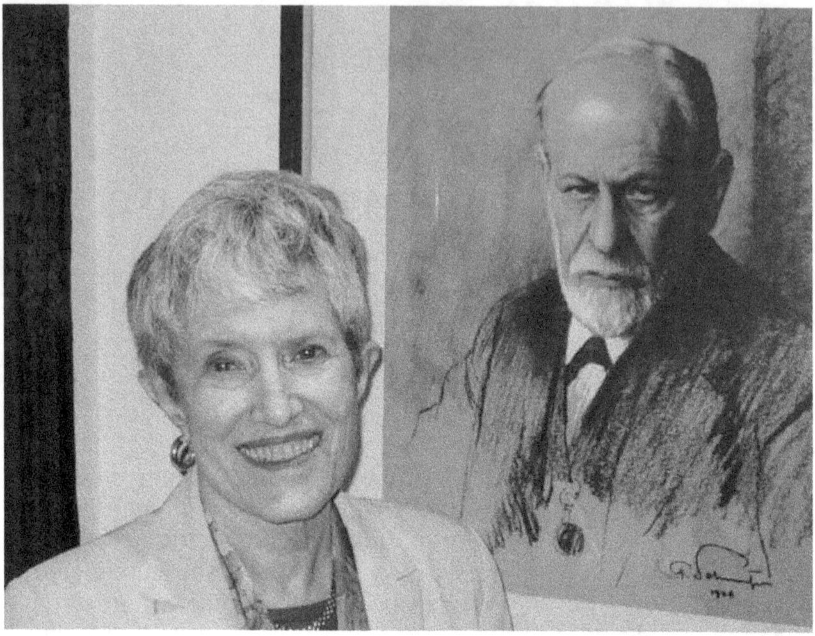

with her long-term partner, Nadia Doubins. Nadia is a Londoner who received her PhD in French Literature from the University of California, Los Angeles (UCLA), and taught in the French Department at Wellesley College. They met in 1981, after Nadia had returned to Los Angeles and was working in administration at UCLA. Drs. Kirkpatrick and Doubins travel extensively and share a love for opera, Native American culture, and modern art. They joyfully play co-grandmothers to Dr. Kirkpatrick's stepson, two sons, and five grandchildren.

Dr. Kirkpatrick was born in Oxnard, California, on December 30, 1925. After spending the first year of life in Los Angeles, she and her mother moved to Battle Creek, Michigan, where John Kellogg had first established his sanitarium and cereal empire. In adolescence, she discovered Freud's writings—sparking a fascination that has never ended. She pursued a BA at the University of Michigan, where she had her first experience with psychotherapy. During a semester at Radcliff College she had the good fortune of taking a psychology seminar with Gordon Allport.[1]

Martha Kirkpatrick applied to Harvard Medical School the first year it accepted women students. Her application was delayed because two alumni interviewers never forwarded their evaluations. Harvard eventually accepted her, but she decided instead to matriculate at McGill Medical School in Montréal and graduated in 1950. Upon returning to her native Los Angeles for internship at the Good Samaritan Hospital, she began the first of five personal psychoanalyses during internship with members of the Los Angeles Psychoanalytic Society and Institute (LAPSI).

Internship provoked a crisis of disillusionment in the medical profession so she spent a summer studying furniture design at the Chouinard Art School. She amusedly recalls that she did not excel at this, even though she has kept herself busy with various design projects over the years.

In 1952, Dr. Kirkpatrick started her residency in psychiatry at the Veteran's Administration Neuropsychiatric Hospital. This was before the introduction of the first antipsychotic, chlorpromazine, in 1954. Psychoanalysis was in its prime, and she fondly recalls being able to spend extensive time with patients without the pressures of brief hospital stays. After completing residency, she launched into private practice in Los Angeles, hoping to be admitted into the LAPSI training program. She was turned down. As a single woman with a history of lesbian relationships, no psychoanalytic program at the time would have accepted her.

In 1957, she married a LAPSI analyst, Seymour Pastron, and had two children, Chipper and Willard. Motherhood was an exciting time, and she recalls having learned much about child development and the dynamics of parenting. Her private practice continued to develop, and she joined the clinical faculty in the UCLA Department of Psychiatry in 1956 (eventually rising to the rank of clinical professor).

Dr. Kirkpatrick's second application to LAPSI was successful, and she began analytic training in 1965. It was a time of heated, sometimes acrimonious, debate between classical and Kleinian analysts. Dr. Kirkpatrick learned from all the schools of thought and avoided any single ideological commitment. She graduated from LAPSI in 1971 and began a private practice in psychoanalysis. In 1988, she joined the faculty of LAPSI and is now a member of the institute's senior faculty. She is also training and supervising analyst at the Institute of Contemporary Psychoanalysis in Los Angeles.

Dr. Kirkpatrick quickly became engaged in various committees at LAPSI as well as in the American Psychiatric Association, the American Academy of Psychoanalysis, and the American Psychoanalytic Association. She also chaired committees of psychiatric and psychoanalytic associations at the local, national, and international levels, particularly dealing with issues concerning children, women, and sexuality. She joined the Group for the Advancement of Psychiatry in 1982, and became chair of its Social Issues Committee in 1992. In 1982 she became a member of the American College of Psychiatrists and was inducted as a fellow in 1990.

Throughout her career, she has also been an active volunteer in a variety of Los Angeles organizations dealing with women's mental health, childhood education, and sex education. From 1985 to 1991 she was on the board of directors of the National Gay Rights Advocates.

In the late 1970s, Dr. Kirkpatrick and two colleagues at UCLA (psychologist Catherine Smith and child psychiatrist Ron Roy) began a comparative study of children of heterosexual versus lesbian mothers. Their results, first presented at the American Psychological Association meeting in 1979, and published in 1981, indicated that the two groups of mothers were quite similar on a variety of measures. The two groups of twenty children also did not differ significantly in the type or frequency of emotional problems. Furthermore, there were no indications that being raised by a lesbian mother had any impact on the gender identity or gender role of children. Like the work of their UCLA colleague, psychologist Evelyn Hooker, their research was part of the first wave of scientific publications arguing against over a century of medical "evidence" for the intrinsic psychopathology of homosexuals and their noxious effects on children.[2]

JGLP: How did you become involved with studying lesbian mothers and their children?

DR. KIRKPATRICK: At the time I started my study of children of lesbian mothers I was a member of Robert Stoller's Gender Identity Clinic at UCLA.[3] We had the opportunity to learn something about the lives, feelings, and frustrations of people with gender dysphoria. We had many occasions to confirm the belief that gender identity, gender role, and sexual orientation ran along different paths and were often contradictory. We saw lots of men and learned a great deal about them, and did what we could to be helpful. We occasionally saw a woman, but very few. I was interested in finding an opportunity to learn something about women's development. It was at the same time—the mid-1970s—that newspapers began reporting on women in court custody battles because of their lesbian relationships. It was clear that neither the judges nor the attorneys nor the women themselves knew what would be the consequences to the children raised in a lesbian household. This was a chance to study how these children were developing. I was particularly interested because I had children of my own—young teenagers at that time. I had also had several passionate lesbian relationships before falling in love with my husband and raising my family. I had often wondered what effect, if any, my lesbian side would have on my children.

In the study of children with lesbian mothers, we discovered many things that were surprising. Since I had lesbian relationships as well as a heterosexual relationship, I thought I would have no presumptions or bias; however, I discovered that I had expected these women to have been coerced into marriage. We found, however, that both the heterosexual and homosexual mothers claimed that, like I, they had married for love of their husband and a desire to have a family. Interestingly enough, although we were not choosing mothers to be alike—we were simply matching children ages five to twelve—the mothers turned out to be quite similar in their pregnancy history, deliveries, and educational and socioeconomic levels.

We discovered some unexpected differences. One of the most impressive was the relationships the children had with their fathers and with men after their mothers had divorced. The children of lesbian mothers had much more contact with their fathers and a great deal more contact with men than the children of divorced, heterosexual mothers. We were mystified by how to explain this but decided it had to do with the heterosexual mothers being much angrier at their husbands and more outraged with the failure of the marriage than had been the lesbian mothers. The lesbian mothers made greater efforts to be sure their children had male companionship since they did not intend to remarry, as perhaps did the heterosexual women.

We also discovered that families moved a great deal more than we expected. In both groups the families moved almost every year! Even when they remained in place, the child care situations could change every few months. We do not know how this instability affects children. We also discovered that the children who had two people in their parenting environment—whatever their age, sex, or relationship—were better off than children with just one parent. They were better off, not just economically, but also socially. They had more social contacts and had more active, richer lives, were more vigorous and broad-minded in their attitudes. It is unclear whether this is the result of having two parental figures or of having the kind of mother who [because she is able to be part of a couple is] more socially adept. It goes against the judgment of some courts in deciding against lesbian mothers in relationships or requiring that the mother must not live with her lesbian lover. From our study, this was clearly not in the best interest of the children.

Another interesting finding was what the children knew about their mother's relationship. Some of the lesbian mothers were very open about their sexual orientation; others were secretive and felt that their children knew nothing about it. From the study, there seemed to be very little relationship between what the mothers thought the children knew and what the children believed. Children who were supposed to know a lot about their mother's lesbianism could still expect her to remarry, while children who were not supposed to know seemed to know a good deal. So we felt that planning in advance for what one should tell one's children remained unclear, since so much seemed to depend on the children's phase of development and their readiness to receive this information.

Overall, we could not find any distinguishing features between the children raised by heterosexual versus lesbian mothers. In both groups, some children had difficulties, but no more in one that the other. Similarly, there were no significant differences in gender disturbances. Our study, like others of the time, looked for proof of difference or no difference between the two groups. As far as I know, all studies based on that aim have been unable to find any identifiable differences in children raised by parents with heterosexual versus homosexual orientations. I hope that in the future there will be studies that instead look at what difference it *does* make to have parents whose sexual orientation deviates from what is socially expected.

JGLP: The social situation has changed much since then. Now there are many lesbian couples having children through artificial insemination or adoption.

DR. KIRKPATRICK: With the ongoing lesbian baby boom, we have many more opportunities to learn how these children will develop, and how they will handle adolescence and their own sexual development.

JGLP: Do you think there is an appropriate time for all children to learn about different sexual orientations, particularly with the gay and lesbian baby boom?

DR. KIRKPATRICK: It seems to me that in the current climate, with more visibility and tolerance (in certain parts of the country) for variations in sexual partnerships and types of family arrangements, that these are questions that should come up and do come up with school-age children. There it can be addressed rather differently than in high school, when the struggle to find one's own identity as a sexual person along with the separation from the parents causes such conflict and intense emotional upheaval.

JGLP: Do you feel it is important for lesbian or gay patients to have gay therapists?

DR. KIRKPATRICK: My usual feeling on this issue is that, to the best one can, one should have a *good* therapist. Hopefully that does not depend on their sexual orientation. From my own experience as a patient and a therapist, I do not have the feeling that the therapist's sexual orientation should be a primary factor in considering a therapist or in making a therapist referral. It reminds me of being asked at an interview for a psychoanalytic institute whether I found it difficult to understand a heterosexual woman. Of course I do not find this difficult. However, it tickled me that I was being asked these questions by a man. I wondered if *he* found it difficult to understand a woman in love with a man, since he had not had this experience himself!

JGLP: In an autobiographical talk you gave at LAPSI on April 25, 2000, you alluded to being rejected initially from training at LAPSI, and that this might have been due to being female and having a lesbian history. Can you talk more about that and other experiences confronting homophobia in analytic circles?

DR. KIRKPATRICK: I recall interviews for analytic training back in the 1950s where it was made very explicit that homosexuality would be a barrier to analytic training on the basis that this was a perversion that was hard to treat and indicated severe pathology. When I first applied for analytic training, I was turned down despite five years of analysis because of my lesbian experiences and my not being manifestly heterosexual. Some years later, after my marriage, I was accepted for training and then completed my training and became a member of the institute. My husband and I divorced some twenty years later, and I began what is now a very long-term lesbian relationship. I was not chastised or dismissed from my institute position, but of course by then there had been a significant shift in attitudes toward homosexuality, and much clear evidence that homosexuality did not necessarily imply the kind of pathology that would make empathy and understanding of heterosexuality impossible.

In more recent times, having had five different analysts in five different analytic experiences, I cannot identify any homophobic point of view. I experienced a great deal of understanding of my homosexual and heterosexual development and an increased sense of tolerance for the intense variability within any person's "sex print," as Ethel Person likes to call it.[4]

JGLP: Does progress still need to be made on gay issues in the analytic community?

DR. KIRKPATRICK: Yes, if progress means full acceptance of homosexual individuals for training. You are probably familiar with the exchange between Freud and Ernest Jones. Jones wrote Freud about a homosexual man who had applied for training in the Dutch psychoanalytic institute. Jones asked for Freud's opinion about rejecting homosexual candidates as a matter of standard policy. Freud's response was that he did not agree. He suggested (as all analysts and institutes should still keep in mind) that an applicant should be considered on the basis of his or her abilities and capacities to be an analyst, not on the basis of one's sexual orientation. That still seems to me to be a wise statement.[5]

JGLP: What has been a greater challenge in your career, facing sexism or homophobia, and how might they be interrelated?

DR. KIRKPATRICK: It is sometimes hard to choose between causes, particularly when you are in a minority position of power in a number of different ways. I have had a very enjoyable political career in the APA, where my identification has been primarily with women's issues and the effort to get more women interested and capable of moving into positions of power at higher levels of governance in the psychiatric profession. I've also tried to maintain contacts and work where I could for gay psychiatrists to feel more at home and have positions of influence as well.

JGLP: How do you feel about the opposing political forces in the community between integration and separatism? Or would you characterize it differently?

DR. KIRKPATRICK: It seems to me that the gay, lesbian, and bisexual committees within the psychiatric and psychological associations are very active and vigorous and have served an important empowerment function for many young gay and lesbian psychiatrists. I imagine that will continue as long as it is necessary to educate the larger community as to the viability and competence of gay and lesbian people. I do tend to prefer, for myself at least, integration to separation. I hope that there will come a time when one can indeed be gay or lesbian and use that in whatever way one likes to understand oneself and others better and to encourage the community to see the value of such diversity. But I hope that we move toward a clear integration with the larger community rather than increased separation.

JGLP: One of the hottest issues now is "gay marriage." How do you feel about it?

DR. KIRKPATRICK: I think one could take a revisionist point of view, as many people seem to, by noting that there are many legal and financial benefits to marriage and that gay couples that are committed should be entitled to receive these benefits. I would rather take a revolutionary position and say that marriage itself has been a failure. That it has not led in our time to the kind of stable family life that can best serve the next generation and, thereby, best generate creative people for our society. I would like to see the whole thing abolished, rather than seeing gay and lesbian people aping an institution that has failed. I have been impressed with the contracts for child care that I have seen coming out of some of the gay and lesbian groups, particularly in San Francisco, where gay and lesbian parents draw up a contract that is aimed at the best interests of the children, rather than seeing them as property. I would like to see that kind of contract used as a model for the heterosexual community, rather than moving toward marriage in its traditional and outmoded form.

JGLP: Much has changed in the United States for lesbians and gays during your lifetime. What do you see as positive developments and which as negative?

DR. KIRKPATRICK: Well, certainly a great deal has changed—changes that can only be viewed as beneficial to the LGB community as well as the larger community. In particular, there is much more support for young people who are discovering their sexuality. There is more support from the regular institutions and much less fear in the workplace and in the community at large, despite the fact that we also know about the hideous stories of prejudicial attacks that continue. A great deal of this change has to be attributed to those who have come forward and been willing to proclaim their positions.

I realize that some of these changes we have to credit to those who have been outrageous in demanding changes. I remember a meeting of the APA in the early 1970s during a discussion of gender identity and role. It was positive toward the gay community, but it was disrupted by some flamboyant activists dressed outrageously. They ran through the audience, grabbed the microphone, and began a discussion of their own point of view. I was angry about this and felt they harmed the cause and were just demonstrating themselves as freaks. However, on the plane home that evening from those meetings—where the American Psychoanalytic Association had decided not to take a stance against the Vietnam War and had eschewed taking a stance on political or social issues altogether—I realized that the only way organizations could be forced to take a position on social issues was if someone was willing to do something outrageous to bring it to their attention. As time went on, I became much more grateful to those who could perform outrageous acts and bring public attention to difficult issues that needed new solutions. I began to wonder why I couldn't do something like that and realized that I was just chicken-shit and couldn't do it! So it seems to me that one should do what one can for the causes one believes in, rather than trying to do what others can do better.

JGLP: Over the years, you have gained extensive clinical experience with a variety of emerging issues of sexuality and sexual orientation. How do you think now about sexuality and ongoing challenges to our understanding of it?

DR. KIRKPATRICK: My own view of sexuality is that it is multilayered, contains a multitude of personal variations, and resembles a kaleidoscope with many flashes of color that shift and change in various circumstances. With this in mind, I hope that the gay and lesbian community will be able to tolerate variations within itself. It is equally hard for gays and lesbians to discover heterosexual parts of themselves as it is for heterosexuals to discover homosexual parts of themselves. I hope that we become more integrated within ourselves, and more accepting of our different impulses and desires, because I feel that helps to bring about a more complete human being.

I have also been struck by the close and valuable friendships between gay men and straight women. I have a number of women friends and patients who have mourned the loss of their close gay friends in the AIDS crisis. It made me aware of the value of those particular relationships. I do not think we have thought much of that in psychiatry, but there is a special kind of a bond in those relationships, and it goes against the old notion that a gay male psychiatrist could never become a great analyst in the treatment of women.

JGLP: What do you think about recent research on the neurobiology or genetics of homosexuality?

DR. KIRKPATRICK: It seems to me that it is highly unlikely that homosexuality is genetically determined. It seems much more multidetermined to me. And I do still very much believe that early fantasy life and the way that personal interactions and family life interact in the psyche play a very important role. I do think, along with Roger Gorski (a neuroanatomist at UCLA), that the brain is a sexual organ, but that it takes the *whole* brain to evolve an individual sexuality.[6] It is not derived through the actions of INAH3 or 4 [hypothalamic nuclei reported to be associated with human sexual orientation].[7]

JGLP: Finally, you and your partner, Nadia Doubins, have been together for twenty years. What is your formula for a long-lasting lesbian relationship?

DR. KIRKPATRICK: *[Laughter]* It goes back to my having twenty years of analysis *previous* to the relationship and, of course, dropping in for a little help whenever one can. There's nothing like knowing yourself for helping you to put up with the strange behaviors that you encounter in yourself and being able to make them work in a relationship.

NOTES

1. Allport was the author of the groundbreaking book *The Nature of Prejudice*. Boston, MA: Beacon, 1954.

2. Hooker, E. (1957), The adjustment of the male overt homosexual. *J. of Projective Techniques,* 21:18-31. Also see Bayer, R. (1987), *Homosexuality and American Psychiatry: The Politics of Diagnosis*. Princeton, NJ: Princeton University Press.

3. Editor's Note: Psychoanalyst Robert Stoller, MD, was a pioneer in the analytic study of sexuality. His publications span the gamut of phenomena that had traditionally been designated "perversions," e.g., homosexuality, transsexualism, transvestitism, and sadomasochism. In the later part of his career—tragically cut short by an accident—he became more skeptical that there was any hard distinction to be made between "normality" and "perversity." Dr. Kirkpatrick is referring to Stoller's work on transsexualism: Stoller, R. J. (1969), *Sex and Gender.* London: Hogarth Press.

4. Person, E. (1980), Sexuality as the mainstay of identity: Psychoanalytic perspectives. *Signs: J. of Women in Culture and Society,* 5:605-630.

5. Editor's Note: On December 1, 1921, Ernest Jones wrote to Freud in Vienna about a query from the Dutch psychoanalytic society concerning the application of a homosexual man to training there. Jones had advised against it; however, he still sought Freud's opinion: "Do you think this would be a safe general maxim to act on?"

Freud replied in a terse letter circulated among the institutes and co-signed by Otto Rank: "Your query, dear Ernest, concerning prospective membership of homosexuals has been considered by us and we disagree with you. In effect we cannot exclude such persons without other sufficient reasons, as we cannot agree with their legal prosecution. We feel that a decision in such cases should depend upon a thorough examination of the other qualities of the candidate" (December 11, 1921).

Jones retorted: "[I]t is hard to see how [homosexuals] could perform a thorough [psychoanalysis] with understanding. Further, our condemnation of the punishment of homosexuality does not alter the fact that to the world it is an abhorrent crime, the committal of which by one of our members would certainly discredit us seriously" (December 21, 1921).

From Berlin, analysts Karl Abraham, Hanns Sachs, and Max Eitington in a circular letter generally agreed with Freud and Rank but had serious reservations: "We have had the experience that homosexuals with an overt behavior pattern can travel only part of the way with us" (January 11, 1922).

Freud and Rank replied: "We recognize the arguments against the analytic participation of homosexuals as somewhat of a guideline. But we have to warn against making it into a law considering the various types of homosexuality and the different mechanisms of their cause" (January 22, 1922).

The correspondence was discovered in the 1970s in the Otto Rank Collection (IIa/238-254) in the Rare Book and Manuscript Library of the Columbia University Libraries. The letters were translated by historian James Steakley and excerpted in: Spiers, H. & Lynch, M. (1977), The gay rights Freud. *Body Politic* (Toronto), 33:8-10. I am grateful to Professor Steakley for corrections and additional material.

6. Allen, L. S. & Gorski, R. A. (1992), Sexual orientation and the size of the anterior commissure in the human brain. *Proc. Nat. Acad. Sci.*, 89:7199-7202.

7. LeVay, S. (1991), A difference in hypothalamic structure between heterosexual and homosexual men. *Science,* 253:1034-1037.

SELECTED BIBLIOGRAPHY

Kirkpatrick, M. (1975), Psychiatry and the women's movement. *Bull. Los Angeles Psychoan. Soc./Inst.* (Spring):76.

Kirkpatrick, M. (1975), A report of a consciousness raising group for women psychiatrists. *J. Amer. Med. Women's Assoc.*, 30:206-212.

Kirkpatrick, M. & Friedman, C. T. (1976), Treatment of requests for sex-change surgery with psychotherapy. *Amer. J. Psychiat.*, 133:1194-1196.

Kirkpatrick, M. (1976), Women's sexual complaints. *Medical Aspects of Human Sexuality,* 10(April):118-125.

Kirkpatrick, M. (1977), Rape: Who cares! *Psychiat. Opinion* (August).

Kirkpatrick, M., contributor (1980), *Human Sexuality: Notes for Physicians.* Board of Medical Quality Assurance, State of California.

Kirkpatrick, M. & Morgan, C. (1980), Psychodynamic psychotherapy of female homosexuality. In: *Homosexual Behavior: A Modern Reappraisal,* ed. Judd Marmor. New York: Basic Books, pp. 357-375.

Kirkpatrick, M., ed. (1980), *Women's Sexual Development.* New York: Plenum.

Kirkpatrick, M., Smith, C. & Roy, R. (1981), Lesbian mothers and their children: A comparative survey. *Am. J. Orthopsychiat.*, 51:545-551.

Kirkpatrick, M., Smith, C. & Roy, R. (1981), Studies of a new population: The lesbian mother. In: *Modern Perspectives in the Psychiatry of Middle Age,* ed. J. G. Howells. New York: Brunner/Mazel, pp. 118-125.

Kirkpatrick, M. (1982), Equality and genitality. *Amer. J. Psychoanal.*, 42:99-107.

Kirkpatrick, M. (1982), Lesbian mother families. *Psychiat. Ann.*, 12:842-848.

Kirkpatrick, M., ed. (1982), *Women's Sexual Experience.* New York: Plenum.

Gottleib, F., Kirkpatrick, M., Marmor, J. & Galanter, M. (1984), Self-help groups. In: *The Psychiatric Therapies,* ed. T. B. Karasu. Washington, DC: American Psychiatric Press, pp. 815-830.

Hitchens, D. & Kirkpatrick, M. (1985), Lesbian mothers/gay fathers. In: *Emerging Issues in Child Psychiatry and the Law,* ed. E. Benedek & D. Schetky. New York: Brunner/Mazel, pp. 115-126.

Kirkpatrick, M. & Miller, D. (1985), Private practice: Springboard or stumbling block for women leaders? In: *Women Physicians in Leadership Roles,* ed. L. & C. Nadelson. Washington, DC: American Psychiatric Press, pp. 185-193.

Kirkpatrick, M. (1987), Book review: *Women, Sexuality and Love* by Georg Simmel. *J. Amer. Psychoanal. Assoc.,* 35:275-279.

Kirkpatrick, M. (1987), Clinical implications of lesbian mothers studies. *J. Homosexuality,* 14(1-2):201-211.

Kirkpatrick, M. (1988), Book review: *Surviving Sexual Contradictions* by Muriel Dimen. *Academy Forum,* 32:20-21.

Kirkpatrick, M. (1988), Some clinical perceptions of middle aged divorcing women. In: *Divorce as a Developmental Process,* ed. J. H. Gold. Washington, DC: American Psychiatric Press, pp. 79-99.

Kirkpatrick, M. (1989), Book review: *Women in Therapy* by H. G. Lerner. *Amer. J. Psychiat.,* 146:271.

Kirkpatrick, M. (1989), Middle age and the lesbian experience. In: *The Middle Years: New Psychoanalytic Perspectives,* ed. J. M. Oldham & R. S. Liebert. New Haven, CT: Yale University Press, pp. 135-148.

Kirkpatrick, M. (1989), Society plays significant role in labeling of women as masochistic. *The Psychiatric Times* (May).

Kirkpatrick, M. (1989), Women in love in the 80's. *J. Amer. Acad. Psychoanal.,* 17:535-542.

Kirkpatrick, M. (1990), Homosexuality and parenting. In: *Women's Progress: Promises and Problems,* eds. J. Spurlock & C. Rabinowitz. New York: Plenum.

Kirkpatrick, M. (1990), Thoughts about the origins of femininity. *J. Amer. Acad. Psychoanal.,* 18:554-565.

Kirkpatrick, M. (1990), Tribute to Nancy C. A. Roeske. In: *Educating Competent and Humane Physicians,* ed. H. C. Hendrie & C. Lloyd. Bloomington, IN: Indiana University Press, pp. x-xi.

Kirkpatrick, M. (1991), Lesbian couples in therapy. *Psychiat. Ann.,* 21:491-496.

Kirkpatrick, M. (1992), Aging, like a woman. In: *How Psychiatrists Look at Aging,* ed. G. Pollock. Madison, CT: International Universities Press, pp. 141-147.

Kirkpatrick, M. (1993), Book review: *Being Homosexual: Gay Men and Their Development* by Richard Isay. *J. Amer. Psychoanal. Assn.,* 41:242-245.

Kirkpatrick, M. (1995), Book review: *Women Analyze Women: In France, England and the United States* by E. H. Baruch & L. J. Seerano. *J. Amer. Psychoanal. Assn.,* 43:1201-1208.

Kirkpatrick, M. (1996), Lesbians as parents. In: *Textbook of Homosexuality and Mental Health,* ed. R. P. Cabaj & T. S. Stein. Washington, DC: American Psychiatric Press, pp. 353-370.

Kirkpatrick, M. & Dickstein L. J. (2000), Women psychiatrists in American postwar psychiatry. In: *American Psychiatry After World War II—1944-1994,* ed.

R. W. Menninger & J. Nemiah. Washington, DC: American Psychiatric Press, pp. 569-593.

Kirkpatrick, M. (2002), The diverse sexuality of lesbians. In: *The Multiple Facets of Lesbianism: Dilemmas and Solutions,* ed. R. S. Fischer & K. Reed. Northvale, NY: Jason Aronson.

Kirkpatrick, M. (2003), The nature and nurture of gender. *Psychoanalytic Inquiry,* 23:558-571.

Chapter 14

An Interview with Richard A. Isay, MD

Robert Mitchell

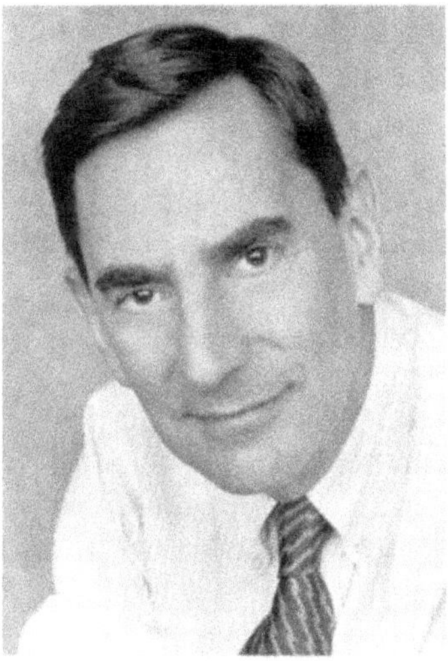

Dr. Richard Isay is known to many as the first openly gay psychoanalyst in the American Psychoanalytic Association (APsaA). Among his many important clinical contributions to psychiatry and psychoanalysis is his developmental theory for male homosexuality, a major revision of the classical psychoanalytic theory. He also played a decisive role in making it possible for openly gay men and women to be accepted for analytic training in the institutes of the APsaA. Dr. Isay attended medical school at the University of Rochester and then did his residency in psychiatry at Yale University. Following two years in the U.S. Navy Medical Corps, he completed psychoanalytic training at the Western New England Institute for Psychoanalysis in New Haven and was on the faculty at Yale until 1981. After moving to New York, he joined the faculty of the Columbia University Center for Psycho-

This chapter appeared originally under the same title in *Journal of Gay & Lesbian Psychotherapy* 6(4):85-96. Copyright 2003 The Haworth Press, Inc.

American Psychiatry and Homosexuality: An Oral History
Published by The Haworth Press, Inc., 2007.
doi:10.1300/6049_15

analytic Training and Research and also joined the faculty at Weill Medical College of Cornell University, where he has been Clinical Professor of Psychiatry since 1989.

Dr. Isay has held a wide variety of leadership positions in major psychoanalytic organizations. He served first as secretary and later chair of the Program Committee for the International Psychoanalytical Association, was president of the Western New England Psychoanalytic Society, and chaired the Program Committee of the APsaA from 1981 until 1984. He also has been chair of the Committee on Gay, Lesbian, and Bisexual Issues of the American Psychiatric Association (APA), vice president of the Board of Directors of the National Lesbian and Gay Health Foundation, a director of the Hetrick-Martin Institute for Gay and Lesbian Youth, and senior consultant to the Columbia University Center for Gay, Lesbian, and Bisexual Mental Health.

Dr. Isay has been a fellow of the APA since 1979. His many awards include the Winfield Scott Award from the National Lesbian and Gay Health Association for outstanding contributions to health care, education, and activism and the Distinguished Service Award from the Association of Gay and Lesbian Psychiatrists.

JGLP: Let me thank you very much for making the time to do this. I want to start by asking about the development of your work with gay men. In your book *Becoming Gay,* you wrote that it was around 1980 that you first started working extensively with gay men. What accounted for that timing?

DR. ISAY: I moved to New York from New Haven in 1980. Then I began to see a lot of gay men who were referred to me after I moved.

JGLP: Did people know you were interested in working with gay men?

DR. ISAY: No, it was coincidence. It was later, around 1983 or 1984, that I began to come out to my gay patients when they inquired about my sexual orientation. It was not only because I thought they needed that information but also because I couldn't do good therapy with gay men feeling that I had this secret. I was out to my wife, but only to her. I found that being concerned that my gay patients might find out in one way or another was considerably detracting from my empathy and my capacity to use my inner resources, my intuition, and my spontaneity in my clinical work. It was keeping my work from being as good as it should have been. Then it became widely known that there was a gay analyst interested in working with gay men and I got many self-referred patients.

JGLP: What made you decide to move to New York then?

DR. ISAY: There were two issues. I was married at the time, and my ex-wife wanted to move and wanted to take a job in the city. The other reason was that I had met Gordon [Dr. Isay's partner]. So both were motives for moving.

JGLP: Soon after that, in 1983, you chaired a great symposium on homosexuality at the winter meeting of the American Psychoanalytic (i.e., APsaA). How did that come about?

DR. ISAY: I had tried for a couple of years to arrange that panel as a member of the program committee. I couldn't get it through. When I became chair of the program committee in 1982, I pushed it through.

JGLP: How much pushing did it take?

DR. ISAY: A lot. It wasn't just a symposium on homosexuality, but on a revision of male homosexuality and on psychoanalytic thinking about homosexuality. Analysts were still very entrenched in old ways of thinking. There was an enormous amount of prejudice and antagonism. But it wasn't simply—and this was a conclusion I came to later—it wasn't simply that they were prejudiced against homosexuals. They felt threatened by and betrayed by any radical innovations or additions to analytic theory.

JGLP: The presentations were terrific. My recollection is that the question-and-answer period seemed incredibly charged. People were very eager to talk, but some people seemed quite disorganized by the experience. Was that your experience?

DR. ISAY: Oh, yes. I remember [Charles] Socarides getting up and he was barely comprehensible. Others walked out.

JGLP: Soon after that symposium, you describe a number of things that must have been disappointing; colleagues stopped sending you referrals; you had a paper rejected by the journal of the APsaA for the first time. What would you describe as your biggest professional disappointments?

DR. ISAY: Between about 1987 and 1991, when I was the only openly gay member of the American Psychoanalytic, a few members whom I knew to be closeted and married stopped having much to do with me. I was more hurt and surprised by that than by the antagonism of the straight analysts. But I've done what I wanted to do. I know I'm a rather independent spirit. I'm opinionated and I don't collaborate especially well. I've spent my days doing my clinical work and have had time to teach and write. I'm very happy with the form my career has taken.

JGLP: How about in terms of being disrespected?

DR. ISAY: I've felt the attitude of the orthodox analytic community was so wrong-headed, biased, and prejudiced that I didn't care much about that. There were a couple of friends that I had when I was married that I lost contact with, and that to some extent still saddens me. But also I found analysts generally, when I was involved in official psychoanalysis, rigid, stiff, rather unimaginative, and ungiving. I believe this was a product of selection thirty years ago, when institutes tended to select obsessional and mildly depressed people, bright but generally not terribly warm. I don't really miss them.

JGLP: Your personal chapter in *Becoming Gay* was very helpful in seeing you in multiple dimensions. The story of your analyst, "Dr. Samuels," seemed particularly powerful to me. You wrote about being in analysis six times a week for several years.

DR. ISAY: For eight years. Then we decreased to five times a week for two years. I was difficult.

JGLP: In your opinion or Dr. Samuels' opinion?

DR. ISAY: Both. We both thought the more often, the more helpful. Now I don't believe that is necessarily true.

JGLP: After you came out, you wrote him and called him and he didn't answer. Did you ever make any more attempts to talk to him?

DR. ISAY: We had breakfast together when I told him I was gay. Then we lost contact. I wrote him again just a few years ago, saying it would be great to get together. He's getting elderly, I wanted to see if he's changed. After about a month, he wrote me back a very formal letter that he could see me at a particular time during the analytic meetings. But the tone of the letter was so frosty that I decided that I didn't want to put myself or him through that. I could just feel the anger and hurt. However, I do remain fond of him. I hope that comes through in the chapter. He did a lot of good things for me;

he's a good person. After my analysis I became friendly with him and his wife and his children. One of the things I didn't put in that chapter is that whenever we had dinner together, he would always have a cigar for me. I hated cigars. I didn't like the taste, but I would light it because he took such pleasure in giving me a cigar to smoke. I remember every time he'd light the cigar for me, I'd take a few puffs, and he'd say, "Atta boy" *[laughs]*. I had that in the chapter, but I took it out because I was afraid it made him look silly and I didn't want to do that. He thought it was manly and masculine, and he did it out of affection.

JGLP: During that decade of your analysis, you had no sex at all with men?

DR. ISAY: As I said in that chapter in my book, I was very caught up in the model: "This is a symptom of something I should get rid of." At that time, I would have been out of the institute if I had said anything else. After we decided on a date for termination, I went a couple of times to a gay book store. We both agreed that it was because I was angry with him for terminating and that it was a manifestation of the transference. That was as close as I came. After we stopped, freed of the analysis, I got very active.

JGLP: You tell the story about almost being arrested [for solicitation] at a Connecticut highway rest stop shortly after that. Did you have any second thoughts about including that episode?

DR. ISAY: No second thoughts about it at all because it was very characteristic of the way married gay men had sex, and the way we put ourselves in harm's way and endangered ourselves and our reputations. It was terrifying and in striking contrast to my being an up-and-coming analyst, a pillar of the community.

JGLP: How did you decide to tell your wife about your being gay?

DR. ISAY: Because I had respect and love for her, I felt that it was appropriate to do so, to give her the opportunity to choose what she wanted to do. But you're taking a risk when you do that, obviously. That's why people choose not to come out to spouses. I was unable to segment my life, and I've never been able to do so. I do not do well with personal secrets.

JGLP: What made you decide to tell her at that point in time?

DR. ISAY: It was 1980, at the time of the psychiatric meetings in San Francisco. I had met Gordon the previous December, so it was about four or five months later. There was a meeting of what was then called the GLB Caucus. Frank Rundle ran it with his lover. And it was right down the hall from where we were staying. After I came back from the meeting, I told her.

JGLP: Was she surprised or had she realized?

DR. ISAY: I don't think she was surprised—partly because of my lack of sexual interest, although she might not have known the details. I found it important for myself and for her to be honest and then let things take their natural course. Our marriage stayed together until the children were old enough to be able to process it. One of the things I heard from both my boys, at the time and subsequently, was that my being gay did not bother them. What bothered them was the image we presented of our having had a happy marriage, which in many ways it was. But they viewed it as sort of a mind-fuck. When they were confronted with the reality of the situation, it caused them to question their perception of reality. The idea of their father being gay, this was not as important an issue. My older son, who is a radio journalist and producer, has made a vocation of his interest in very different, unconventional people, and my younger son, a political consultant, will only work with candidates who are social liberals.

JGLP: There were two big political contributions you made in terms of the American Psychoanalytic. Around 1989 you got them to say that homosexuality was not an illness and to begin admitting gay candidates.

DR. ISAY: I had asked the Board of Professional Standards [of the APsaA] to pass the nondiscrimination statement that the APsaA had passed in 1973. They refused on a couple of occasions. So I went to *Psychiatric News* [the monthly newsletter of the American Psychiatric Association] with the story. The publicity then forced the Board of Professional Standards to pass the statement. They did not want to be seen as prejudiced against homosexuals. They were very angry about my having done that, insisting that there never was any prejudice or bias in the APsaA.

JGLP: Then you took a more provocative step with the threat of a lawsuit.

DR. ISAY: That was occasioned by their refusal to approve homosexuals as training analysts. I had sent a letter asking the Board of Professional Standards to state explicitly that homosexuals could be training analysts, which they did not want to do. I can't remember whether they refused to take up the issue or outright rejected the motion.

JGLP: So you got the American Civil Liberties Union (ACLU) to threaten a lawsuit.

DR. ISAY: Yes. Then the association acted very quickly. Within two weeks, the American Psychoanalytic had a very explicit statement to the effect that homosexuals could be training analysts.

JGLP: Then within a few years, the American Psychoanalytic seemed to become more progressive.

DR. ISAY: There continues to be a gradually changing, more accepting view of gays and lesbians.

JGLP: The American Psychoanalytic came out in favor of same-sex unions at least two years earlier than the American Psychiatric Association did.

DR. ISAY: Yes, and I think it's good and appropriate that they did. But like any orthodoxy, there is still a good deal of hypocrisy in institutional classical psychoanalysis, which will hopefully change as organized psychoanalysis continues to become more diverse.

JGLP: Has the American Psychoanalytic taken a position on reparative therapy?

DR. ISAY: They do have a statement to the effect that psychoanalysis should not try to effect such change, but they always had maintained that psychoanalysis properly practiced does not encourage or coerce anyone to change any behavior. In general, they do not like to acknowledge the coercive or suggestive nature of analysis. But traditional psychoanalysts did try, some indirectly and some in explicit ways, to encourage change of sexual orientation. My analyst never said to me, "You should change from homosexual to heterosexual." But he also never said to me, "Have you thought that you might be homosexual?" Essentially, he unconsciously used my transference need for his love to attempt to change me.

JGLP: You must be very proud of the political work that you've accomplished.

DR. ISAY: Yes, I'm proud of it, but I worry a bit about this. I have some questions about what the gay candidates who are in training now are going to do with their training. Most want analytic training to learn to be good psychotherapists. But I am not sure this is the best training for anyone at the present time. Traditional four-times-a-week, on-the-couch analysis, I feel, has always been a better investigative tool than a therapy. There aren't a lot of people being psychoanalyzed now, and interest in psychoanalytic training is not as great as it once was. This lack of interest in training has contributed to the eagerness of analytic institutes to accept gay candidates, psychologists, and social workers. There's nothing wrong with that. It's good for psychoanalysis to have a broad, diverse group of candidates. It will change the technique and make it a better treatment.

JGLP: And helpful to a lot of potential candidates who otherwise might have been denied training. How many openly gay training analysts are there now?

DR. ISAY: I'm not sure.

JGLP: It's something you decided not to go for.

DR. ISAY: Yes. There was a time in the early 1980s when I was beginning to write about gay men that I thought it would be helpful to be a training analyst. I was told I was on the "track" but that I would have to spend much more time on committees of the local analytic institute and be more of a team player.

JGLP: You've been a very good team player in the past, but it seems as you talk about it now that you like the role of rebel more. Is that correct?

DR. ISAY: It was an adaptation to the position I was in. If I was married, living as a heterosexual, knowing that I wasn't, then I might as well do a good job with all of it. So I wrote very boring but acceptable papers for the *Journal of the American Psychoanalytic Association,* was early on a member of the faculty of the Western New England Institute and their board of trustees, and on important committees of the American and International Psychoanalytic Associations.

JGLP: You were president of the Western New England Institute at quite a young age.

DR. ISAY: A couple of years after I finished training. I was also considered in the early 1980s, albeit very briefly, as a possible candidate for president of the American Psychoanalytic. I adapted well to my heterosexual life on the outside, but I was always feeling "different," very anxious and angry.

JGLP: You've been in a relationship with Gordon for two decades. How do you do that?

DR. ISAY: It will be twenty-three years in December 2002. He's a lovely, wonderful man. We were both committed to the relationship and to each other from very early on. It's the commitment that makes it possible to take each other's needs into account, to be willing to be dependent on each other. The bottom line is that he's a terrific guy. There's no one I enjoy being with as much or whom I find as smart and funny. We love and care about each other.

JGLP: Do you think a long-term relationship is desirable for most gay men, or do you think they need a wider variety of options?

DR. ISAY: I do think it's desirable. The stability and love are essential for happiness. There are difficulties imposed by society and early developmental issues that make it problematic for some to have a stable, loving relationship. Many gay men, and heterosexuals, too, are not willing to make the compromises that a relationship entails. But the difficulty some gay men have with intimacy causes too many not to want a relationship that extends over a long period of time, or to prefer friends, periodic sexual encounters, or "extended family" as substitutes for the love of one person.

JGLP: You wrote that at one point in your analysis you no longer felt passion.

DR. ISAY: That was when I entered into analysis. Passion was kept in check by my attempts to be heterosexual. I rediscovered my passion when I rediscovered my homosexuality. In a recent paper, I wrote indirectly about passion. There are a lot of gay men who are out and self-acknowledged who have disavowed the feminine aspect of themselves and, in the process, have also given up their passion, their expressiveness, and their dependence, all of which are important in intimate, romantic, long-term relationships. Many divert a lot of their passion into random sexual encounters instead, which can be exciting and fun, but they're also the enemy of intimacy.

JGLP: What do you think are good solutions for those gay people for whom their religion is very important and where that religion explicitly prohibits homosexual behaviors?

DR. ISAY: I treated one priest, a conservative Catholic theologian. He had the most amazing logical ways of rationalizing his behavior. I learned from him that one can stay devout and still find ways to live the kind of life that you're comfortable living. About six or seven years ago, I spoke at a large meeting of Catholics known as the New Ways Ministry. There were perhaps 700 people attending, who were trying to reconcile Catholic dogma with what they hear in church and see in their own lives. I was very impressed by the group, by how devout they were and how many were intent on trying to find a way to bring together these disparate aspects of their lives. I have been concerned about some of my patients who have been brought up in devout families who have been so alienated that they have given up traditions that were important to them and connections with family that had been important. I don't think religion or tradition necessarily has to be tossed out. I think our lives are richer at times by trying to bring contradictions together.

JGLP: What are you currently working on professionally?

DR. ISAY: I have a good draft of a new book. Both of the previous books were given as papers. This one I wanted to do more as a book and write it all together, rather than as separate papers, so the process is a bit different. I think it's an interesting and important book and that it will be helpful, though it will be controversial. I don't enjoy the process of writing. I spend a couple of hours Saturday morning and a couple hours Sunday morning. It's a very long, drawn-out process for me. It takes forever. I've been working on this book for a couple of years.

JGLP: Where does your current thinking differ from that of twenty-five years ago?

DR. ISAY: Clinically, I'm much more interactive with my patients and more giving. Hopefully I'm not being oblivious to the enactments that are occurring. But the idea that one cannot answer questions and be interactive and still understand what's on the patient's mind is a myth. I think it's the intent of what one is saying and the care and concern of the therapist that patients respond to. The therapist's "love" is much more important to the therapeutic process than I thought twenty-five years ago.

SELECTED BIBLIOGRAPHY

Isay, R. (1968), The submariners' wives syndrome. *Psych. Quart.,* 42:647-652.

Isay, R. (1968), The draft-age adolescent in treatment. *Psych. Quart.,* 43:203-210.

Isay, R. (1975), The influence of the primal scene on the sexual behavior of the early adolescent. *J. Amer. Psychoan. Assn.,* 23:535-553.

Isay, R. (1977), Ambiguity in speech. *J. Amer. Psychoan. Assn.,* 25:427-452.

Isay, R. (1978), The pathogenicity of the primal scene. *J. Amer. Psychoan. Assn.,* 26:131-142.

Isay, R. (1981), Late adolescence: The second separation stage of adolescence. In: *The Course of Life,* Volume 2, ed. S. Greenspan & G. Pollock. Adelphi, MD: Mental Health Study Center, NIMH, pp. 511-522.

Isay, R. (1985), On the analytic therapy of homosexual men. *The Psychoanalytic Study of the Child,* 40:235-254. New Haven, CT: Yale University Press.

Isay, R. (1986), The development of sexual identity in homosexual men. *The Psychoanalytic Study of the Child,* 41:467-489. New Haven, CT: Yale University Press.

Isay, R. (1987), Fathers and their homosexually inclined sons in childhood. *The Psychoanalytic Study of the Child,* 42:275-294. New Haven, CT: Yale University Press.

Isay, R. (1988), Homosexuality in homosexual and heterosexual men: Some distinctions and implications for treatment. *Psych. Annals,* 18:43-46.

Isay, R. (1989), *Being Homosexual: Gay Men and Their Development.* New York: Farrar, Straus and Giroux.

Isay, R. (1990), Psychoanalytic theory and therapy of gay men. In: *Homosexuality/Heterosexuality: Concepts of Sexual Orientation,* ed. D. McWhirter, S. Sanders, & J. Reinisch. New York: Oxford University Press, pp. 293-303.

Isay, R. (1993), Dynamic psychotherapy with gay men: Developmental considerations. *Review of Psychiatry,* 12:85-100. Washington, DC: American Psychiatric Press.

Isay, R. (1993), The homosexual analyst: Clinical considerations. In: *Affirmative Dynamic Psychotherapy with Gay Men,* ed. C. Cornett. Northvale, NJ: Jason Aronson, pp. 177-198.

Isay, R. (1996), *Becoming Gay: The Journey to Self-Acceptance.* New York: Pantheon Books.

Isay, R. (1998), Heterosexually-married homosexual men: Clinical and developmental issues. *Amer. J. Orthopsych.,* 68:424-432.

Isay, R. (1999), Gender in homosexual boys. *Psychiatry: Interpersonal and Biological Process,* 62:187-194.

Chapter 15

An Interview with Richard C. Pillard, MD

Paul E. Lynch

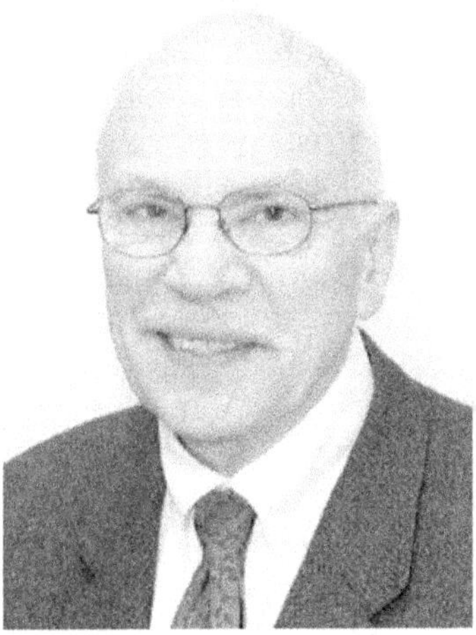

Richard C. Pillard, MD, is Professor of Psychiatry at Boston University School of Medicine and perhaps is best known for studying the incidence of homosexuality in families and twins, and reporting the evidence for genetic heritability. Dr. Pillard has authored about 100 book chapters, articles, reviews, posters, and editorials on psychopharmacology, sexual orientation, and the genetics of deafness. He was also the founder of one of the first gay-oriented health services in the country: The Homophile Community Health Service in Boston, Massachusetts. In addition to clinical work and research, Dr. Pillard spent eight years in administration, as Medical Director and Associate Superintendent for Clinical Services, Dr. Solomon Carter Fuller Mental Health Center in Boston. Recently he took a year to visit Paris and is now back in Boston seeing clinic patients part-time. As he describes in this interview, Dr. Pillard believes he is living the life that his father would have enjoyed.

This chapter appeared originally under the same title in *Journal of Gay & Lesbian Psychotherapy* 7(4):63-70. Copyright 2003 The Haworth Press, Inc.

American Psychiatry and Homosexuality: An Oral History
Published by The Haworth Press, Inc., 2007. All rights reserved.
doi:10.1300/6049_16

JGLP: This year we are celebrating the thirtieth anniversary of the American Psychiatric Association's (APA) removal of homosexuality from the *Diagnostic and Statistical Manual*'s (DSM) list of illnesses. Were you present for the controversial meetings that were disrupted by gay activists, or the one in which John Fryer spoke as Dr. H. Anonymous?[1]

DR. PILLARD: I was not present, but heard about them from friends and fellow psychiatrists. The part that some people do not know is that John Fryer was the official organist of the APA. At the annual meetings, he played the organ to start the session.

The 1960s were all about demonstrations, so perhaps it's not surprising that the demonstrators made their way to the 1970 APA meeting in San Francisco. The old guard psychiatrists (Bieber, Socarides, and others) were presenting papers about how homosexuality could be "cured" by psychotherapy. Gay infiltrators began yelling from the audience and the psychiatrists on stage began yelling back. The psychiatrists' vitriol was shocking. To many in the audience it revealed a kind of organic hatred toward gays that was very inappropriate—the more so if indeed they were mentally ill, as the panelists were claiming. A moderate contingent understood this. From there things unfolded. Dr. Frank Kameny (an astronomer and gay activist) spoke later at an a APA meeting in Washington, DC, and his comments were so clear and straightforward that reasonable psychiatrists began to take notice.

JGLP: Were you out at the time of these controversial meetings? I know that somewhere along the line you were married and had children.

DR. PILLARD: I came out in 1967, after my psychoanalysis with Dr. Sam Silverman. That was a powerful analytic experience. I didn't have any agenda about gayness in the beginning, but as the analysis proceeded, I found myself to be feeling more and more sexual interest in men.

JGLP: How did Dr. Silverman handle that?

DR. PILLARD: Well, he was analytically neutral. He never said anything directly negative or positive about it to me. Years later, I saw an article in the *National Enquirer,* of all places, and it quoted a Dr. Sam Silverman from Boston making all kinds of extremely homophobic statements. I wondered if it could be the same person. How many psychiatrists with that name could there be in Boston? Anyway, he was very helpful to me personally, and I do think the analysis allowed me to come out, and do so with minimal fears or conflicts. There really is something to analysis . . . as you might have noticed.

JGLP: How did your coming out and that period of change in psychiatry affect your career?

DR. PILLARD: Well, Robert Spitzer and J. D. Rosenham were opening up debate at the time about whether psychiatry could distinguish illness from a behavior that was simply eccentric or unpopular. Psychiatrists were waking up to the idea that homosexuality was considered an illness only because of our Western ethnocentric bias. That decision removed the obligation of psychiatrists to treat all gay people as ill and for gay psychiatrists to remain closeted. Before long, we were the largest caucus in the American Psychiatric Association, and, of course, we threw the best parties at the annual meeting!

Today, being a gay psychiatrist is virtually a mainstream experience. I think the profession, to its credit, soaked us up without a hiccup. The DSM diagnostic revision also empowered gay and lesbian patients both to confront psychiatrists as well as to trust them. The downside is that colleagues sometimes expect us to be experts on gay issues just because we are gay.

JGLP: What was it like for you locally? Were there factors that made it possible for you to come out professionally in Boston, and in your department at Boston University?

DR. PILLARD: I was fortunate to be working in the research lab of Dr. Seymour Fischer, a wonderful mentor who didn't care who was gay and who wasn't. Therefore, I didn't worry about my position there.

JGLP: Was there anyone in particular who influenced your coming out as a psychiatrist?

DR. PILLARD: I'm grateful to the late Dr. Howard Brown, then the Commissioner of Health for New York City and the first physician to come out publicly.[2] He did it at age fifty-four after suffering a heart attack and realizing he might not have long to live. His coming out made the front page of the *New York Times*. I was eager to meet him and found him to be a wonderfully bright, lively, interesting, and warm-hearted man. A few months later, he was asked to appear in an article in *Medical World News*. He asked a few of us who he knew were out if we wanted to appear with him in the article. I demurred only a second before saying "yes." So I became the first publicly identified gay psychiatrist. This would have been in 1971 or 1972. Howard died shortly after and I've always been sorry he couldn't have lived to see what he pioneered.

JGLP: Would you discuss your founding of the Homophile Community Health Service, and describe what that experience was like?

DR. PILLARD: The Homophile Community Health Service was founded in 1971 and lasted about ten years. I think it was the first gay-oriented health service in the country. I founded it with Reverend Don McGaw, who continues to practice in Boston, and three other therapists. It was a voluntary agency, a child of the 1960s. We scrounged a place to see patients and were successful in getting a salary block from the state. It was a significant organization in its day—though we always struggled to survive. Eventually, the Fenway Community Health Center emerged as the place for gay people to go for medical care, and their counseling and psychiatric services grew to be more sophisticated.

JGLP: Who were the patients of the Homophile Community Health Service, and what kind of services did you provide?

DR. PILLARD: Basic psychiatric and counseling services for the range of symptoms: anxiety, depression, adjustment problems. The patients who came were generally younger, the first flush of post-Stonewall's openly gay men and lesbians. It was important to give support to people who were being oppressed because they couldn't—or didn't want to—pass for straight.

JGLP: The Homophile Community Health Service must have been a colorful place.

DR. PILLARD: Yes, and very inspiring too. I think we owe a debt to the people who led the gay movement. They weren't congressmen or professors. The courageous early leaders of the gay movement were ordinary working people—shipping clerks, elevator operators, hairdressers, and the unemployed. They had to be tough to survive, and rather than hide they developed this attitude of "Don't mess with a sissy." The Mattachine Society, which existed here in Boston in the 1960s, was made up largely of working-class people.[3]

JGLP: How did you get involved in the research of gayness in families?

DR. PILLARD: I always was involved in research. Initially it was psychopharmacology, and in the late 1970s I had my own lab where I did the family research. Looking at my own family, I wondered if the clustering of gay people in families was more typical than generally realized. The results were compelling. We found that 20 percent of the brothers of gay men were also gay, while only 3 percent of the brothers of straight men were gay.

J. Michael Bailey planned a twin study comparing sexual orientation in identical versus fraternal twins. He's a psychologist with a background in math. The study results showed evidence of a heritable component for being a gay man, less so for being a lesbian. I think female sexual orientation is more variable than is male. Men seem more often to be fixed from early adolescence, even from early childhood. There is still a lot of research to do there, but administrative work at the Fuller took over my interest, and that research still waits to be pursued.

JGLP: What was your own family background like, and how did your family get you interested in research on the heritability of gayness?

DR. PILLARD: My father was an English professor at Antioch College in Ohio, which is where I grew up. I believe that he was a gay man. When he was living as a bachelor in New York City, he was involved in a sailing accident in which his two best friends were drowned. I've always suspected that one of them was his lover. After the accident, he became a Roman Catholic, married in his mid-thirties, and had three children—all gay. My siblings came to it earlier than I did—I was the slow learner who got married. My father died when I was twenty-five, so he wasn't around when my gay life started in my thirties. I never got to tell him about it. My mother said she didn't see any sign of his being gay, but a close friend of my father's told me that he acknowledged having had a gay relationship. At that time, being even suspected of gay tendencies ruined one's career. There was an article recently in the *Harvard Magazine* about several students kicked out of Harvard years ago because they were suspected to be homosexual. Their careers were destroyed and one of them committed suicide. That was around the same time that my father and his friends—theater people like Cole Porter—were at Yale.

JGLP: You have two siblings, and all three of you are gay?

DR. PILLARD: Yes. My brother had the worst of it, really. He was more stereotypically gay, and also very much overweight, which made him self-conscious and shy. He was a likable man but lived an isolated life. I feel guilty of making it worse for him—ridiculing and teasing him. He was a sensitive gay man, and I picked on him a fair amount. But when I came out, I turned to him and he was very kind. He died in his sleep in his fifties. My sister is doing well. She knew she was a lesbian early on and she made an excellent adaptation. She lives with her lover now in Reno where she is a retired professor of social work. By coincidence, her interest is sex research too; she publishes motives for women entering and leaving prostitution. We see each other whenever we can.

JGLP: What was your mother like, and how did she figure in this gay family?

DR. PILLARD: My mother came from a large Baltimore working-class family. She worked her way through college, the only one of five siblings who got that far. Later in her life, she had no knowledge of gayness and it was embarrassing to her that all her children were "like that." One of her sisters had a daughter, my cousin, who was lesbian. My mother told me about an unmarried uncle who lived in her parents' home with a male "friend." It just never occurred to anyone back then that those two might be gay, but now of course it is obvious that all the signs were there.

JGLP: You said you were the slow learner who got married. How did that come about?

DR. PILLARD: I went to Swarthmore, mostly to get out of Yellow Springs, Ohio, but I hated Swarthmore. I transferred back to Antioch, which had a work-study program, so I could travel and live around the country. I went to medical school at the University of Rochester, and it was during medical school in 1958 that I got married. My wife was a Vassar student. The internship/residency computer match matched me with Boston City Hospital for my internship. I stayed at Boston University for my psychiatry residency. It was while I was a resident, around 1963 or so, that I got into analysis.

JGLP: How is it that you got into analysis?

DR. PILLARD: I had always wanted to be analyzed. For an aspiring psychiatrist, it seemed a natural thing to do. I wonder how different life might be if I'd spent the time and money on a vacation, or a hot stock, or whatever. In the end, I think it was an important investment for me.

JGLP: You said that the analysis helped you to come out unafraid.

DR. PILLARD: That's true. I came out after I got divorced. The divorce was quite painful. I was in my thirties by then and it was tough leaving the kids. We didn't get divorced because I was gay—we just weren't getting along. I had a girlfriend after the divorce; it took me another year to come out. I wanted to stay in Boston to be close to my kids. In some ways, I feel I've got the best of the straight world and the best of the gay world. I'm pleased to see gay people adopting kids and mothering/fathering kids and establishing families. It's been a great experience for me to be a father, and I think it's an amazing social development to see gay people as parents.

JGLP: Since you left your wife, you've had gay partners. Did you include them in your professional life, for example, the psychiatry department parties or other functions?

DR. PILLARD: No, not really. My partners were generally younger, so it might have been awkward—though my colleagues were really quite supportive. I'm not planning to live with anyone again, at least not until I'm old and feeble. I'm not there yet, but you never know.

JGLP: You are still involved in research?

DR. PILLARD: Yes, with a psycholinguist friend, Harlan Lane, a Macarthur Award winner. We're studying New England families where there is hereditary deafness. A French abbot first brought deaf people together in Paris and allowed them to develop sign, their natural language. In the early 1800s, a deaf student of the abbot, Laurent Clair, founded the first school for the deaf in Hartford. For our project, Harlan and I examine school records, census records, family genealogies, etc., to learn how deafness travels through the generations. Some of the first deaf families arrived on Martha's Vineyard in the early 1700s. A few of these Vineyard pioneers traveled to Maine, and that's where we are focusing now. Basically, we're reconstructing the heritage of the deaf, their family trees, their language, and their ethnicity. Of interest to me is that many more deaf men seem to be gay than the luck of the draw would predict.

JGLP: Do you have ideas about why?

DR. PILLARD: Well, I have a theory for everything. Probably most of us have some capacity for both homosexual and heterosexual pleasure, but by the time we are beyond our twenties, we tend to be fairly exclusively either gay or straight, much less often bisexual. I tend to think that sexual orientation is influenced by brain organization, that it's more biological, at least for men.

The language of those born profoundly deaf is sign, a spatial language. Learning sign might produce subtle changes in brain localization of certain cognitive functions that could make a gay orientation more likely. People who work with the deaf estimate that perhaps 10 or 15 percent of genetically deaf men are gay versus only 3 or 4 percent of the general population. In short, I think the biology of gayness and of deafness are related.

JGLP: Are you very much involved in the Boston University Psychiatry Department these days?

DR. PILLARD: I still teach there occasionally. I've had my fill of administration and now I like to do what doctors should do—see patients. I never tire of seeing patients; there is always something fascinating to learn. You have a privileged insight into human nature. Since I've been back to work, after a year living in Paris, I've been working at two clinics part-time. It's just about right for me.

JGLP: What were you doing in Paris?

DR. PILLARD: I had a wonderful year, eating, drinking, seeing the sights, visiting friends, and trying to learn French. Learning a language as an adult is a lot harder than when you are young. Once, after I'd made yet another blunder in French class, my teacher asked, incredulously, "Are you really a professor in the States?" Alas, I am.

It occurred to me that living in Paris is one of the things that my father had always wanted to do. He visited Paris in the Roaring Twenties but never lived there. I felt that I had the chance to live a chapter of life that he would have liked—but in his circumstance, it was not possible. I've been blessed to live as an openly gay man, to have loving gay relationships, to enjoy the things that he would have enjoyed—including a year in gay Paris.

JGLP: That's wonderful! I have really enjoyed talking with you today. Merci for your contributions to the field of psychiatry and to the gay and lesbian community. Thank you also for spending this time with me and discussing this interesting and valuable history.

DR. PILLARD: You're welcome.

NOTES

1. Editor's Note: See Bayer, R. (1981), *Homosexuality and American Psychiatry: The Politics of Diagnosis*. New York: Basic Books; and David Scasta's article on John E. Fryer, MD, and the Dr. H. Anonymous episode, Chapter 1 in this book.

2. Editor's Note: See Brown, H. (1976), *Familiar Faces, Hidden Lives: The Story of Homosexual Men in America Today*. New York: Harcourt, Brace Jovanovich.

3. "Founded in 1950 . . . the [Mattachine] Society saw as its primary function the full integration of homosexuals into American life. Concerned with discrimination in employment, the exclusion of homosexuals from the mainstream of social life, and the threat of criminal sanctions against those who engaged in sexual activity in private, [Mattachine] sought to dispel the image of the morally depraved pervert incapable of assuming conventional roles. It cultivated an aura of respectability and propriety, seeking the support of theologians, lawyers, scientists, and psychiatrists in the struggle for the acceptance of homosexuals" (Bayer, *Homosexuality and American Psychiatry*, p. 70).

SELECTED BIBLIOGRAPHY

Pillard, R. C., Poumadere, J. & Carretta, R. A. (1982), A family study of sexual orientation. *Archives of Sexual Behavior*, 11:411-420.

Pillard, R. C. & Weinrich, J. D. (1986), Evidence of familial nature of male homosexuality. *Archives of General Psychiatry*, 43:808-812.

Bailey, J. M., Pillard, R. C., Neale, M. C. & Agyei, Y. (1993), Heritable factors influence sexual orientation in women. *Archives of General Psychiatry*, 50:217-223.

Pillard, R. C. (1996), Homosexuality from a familial and genetic perspective. In: *Homosexuality and Mental Health: A Comprehensive Textbook*, ed. R. P. Cabaj & T. S. Stein. Washington, DC: American Psychiatric Press, pp. 115-128.

Pillard, R. C. (1997), The search for a genetic influence in sexual orientation. In: *Science and Homosexualities*, ed. V. Rosario. New York: Routledge, pp. 226-241.

Pillard, R. C. & Bailey, J. M. (1998), Human sexual orientation has a heritable component. *Human Biology*, 70:343-361.

Lane, H., Pillard, R. C. & French, M. (2002), Origins of the American deaf world. In: *Progress in Sign Language Research*, ed. R. Schulmeister & H. Reinitzer. Hamburg, Germany: Signum-Verlag, pp. 11-30.

Chapter 16

An Interview with Edward Hanin, MD

Jack Drescher

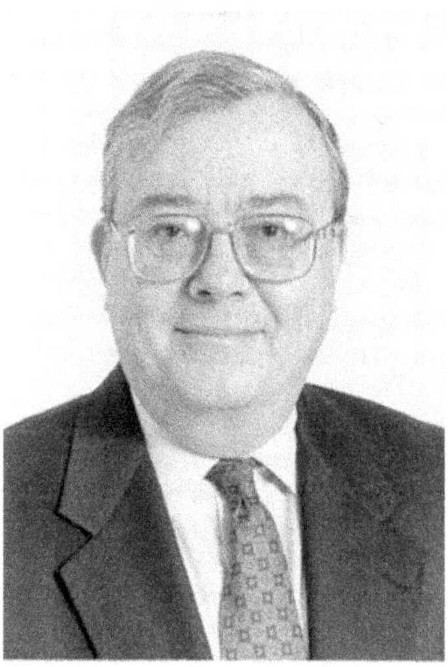

Edward Hanin, MD, a member of the Association for Gay and Lesbian Psychiatrists (AGLP), has had an outstanding and distinguished career in American psychiatry, and particularly within the American Psychiatric Association (APA) where he has served in many important positions. He was President (1978-1979) of the Westchester District Branch (DB) of the APA and later that DB's Representative to the APA Assembly (1981-1984). He was Vice President (1984-1986) and then President (1986-1988) of the New York State Psychiatric Association, simultaneously serving as the Deputy Area Representative to the APA Assembly from New York State (Area II), then Area II's Representative to the APA Assembly. He was later elected by the APA Assembly to be its Recorder (1988-1989) and then Speaker of the Assembly (1990-1991). He chaired APA's Council on National Affairs

This chapter appeared originally under the same title in *Journal of Gay & Lesbian Psychotherapy* 6(2):87-97. Copyright 1998 The Haworth Press, Inc.

doi:10.1300/6049_17

(1996-1999), the Psychiatric News Editorial Advisory Board (1991-2000), and the Joint Commission on National Affairs (1991-1994).

Dr. Hanin has been Clinical Professor of Psychiatry at New York Medical College since 1982. Among his many professional associations, he is Fellow of the American College of Psychiatrists and the New York Academy of Medicine. He is also a member of the Group for the Advancement of Psychiatry. He has been the recipient of numerous professional awards, including the New York State Psychiatric Association's George L. Ginsberg, MD Award (1992), the APA Assembly's Award for Meritorious Service (1995), and the APA's Warren Williams, MD Award (1998).

Dr. Hanin was born in China, a fact of his life which he refers to as "somewhat unusual." His parents were Americans whose family business in China was in Tianjin, the foreign entry port for Beijing. Dr. Hanin came to the United States when he was a year and a half old; he lived in New York City for a while, then in Miami Beach, Florida, then in San Francisco, where he went to junior high school. He returned to New York City where he went to high school, then later attended New York's City College, and then went to New York University Medical School.

After completing his internship and residency in psychiatry at St. Vincent's Medical Center in New York City (1958-1962), Dr. Hanin spent the next two years serving in the U.S. Army. His tour of duty took place during the Cuban Missile Crisis, which he describes as "a very frightening time because I don't think people really recognize how close we were to going to war at that particular point in time." In 1964, he returned to St. Vincent's Hospital where he eventually became the Director of Residency Training and the head of the outpatient clinic. In 1973, he became Chief of Psychiatry at the Westchester branch of St. Vincent's in Harrison, New York. He remained there, directing a 130-bed psychiatric hospital, for about twenty years, until his retirement from the hospital in 1992. He briefly came out of retirement in 1996 to serve as Interim Vice Chairman of St. Vincent's Department of Psychiatry in New York City. Nevertheless, despite his retirement from hospital activity, he maintains an active role within APA governance.

JGLP: Could tell me how you decided to become a psychiatrist?

DR. HANIN: Well, I'm not exactly sure. I'm old enough to have taken what was known as a rotating internship, where you're not forced to make a decision as to your ultimate career choice until after its completion. I really was quite torn between internal medicine and psychiatry, although I did not go to medical school with the idea of going into psychiatry. I went with the idea of just doing medicine.

During my last year in medical school, I had taken an elective in psychiatry at St. Vincent's Hospital in New York City, where I ultimately trained. St. Vincent's was just so different from my previous experience with psychiatry—which up to then had been at Bellevue. At that time, Bellevue was the major receiving hospital for New York City, so the wards were absolutely filled with patients' beds on top of other beds—there was no place to put them and patients would sleep in the hallways. It was a real pit! So I went to St. Vincent's, which had just opened a new psychiatric service, and saw people treated humanely and rationally in a general hospital setting. It was a real eye-opener. During that year as an intern, despite opportunities to pin a hip and do other things, I decided on a career choice in psychiatry and stayed to do my residency training at St. Vincent's.

JGLP: Was there someone at St. Vincent's who drew you to do your training there?

DR. HANIN: Well, there were two people who I would say were significant in that choice. One was the then director of psychiatry, a man by the name of Harvey Tompkins, who had been the director of psychiatry at the VA [Veterans Affairs] before coming to St. Vincent's as its first chair of psychiatry in 1956. As a number of my interests related to administrative matters, seeing someone who was as clinically solid as Tompkins was a real experience. He was a leading figure in psychiatry, very active in the APA, a former obstetrician, and a really interesting man.

Before Tompkins came to St. Vincent's in 1956, its psychiatric section, the Reiss Pavilion, had been originally scheduled to be built a number of years earlier. Just as they were getting going with the pavilion, Monsignor Fulton J. Sheen, in one of his television broadcasts, came out and blasted psychiatry. He said that people who were in trouble should go to their ministers, priests, or rabbis—not to psychiatrists. Well, that created a certain amount of concern at St. Vincent's Hospital. The director of psychiatry at that time, a very distinguished psychiatrist by the name of Frank Curran, spoke out in opposition to Sheen's view of psychiatry. Very shortly thereafter, he was no longer director of psychiatry at St. Vincent's Hospital, and the construction of the Reiss Pavilion was delayed about five years until they brought Dr. Tompkins on board. I was a lowly intern at that point, so I really don't know how or why they changed their minds. But I figure it was just that Dr. Tompkins was a very distinguished Catholic physician, as well as a psychiatrist. And I think he, through a lot of political and educational work, brought people around. He was the one who taught me that just because an idea is a good one, it doesn't automatically happen. There's a fair amount of work that may have to go into preparing the way.

The other person who helped me decide on training at St. Vincent's was Robert J. Campbell, who was then the director of training. He was one of the finest teachers and lecturers that I've ever known in all my years of experience. The number of years that have passed since I was a trainee have not dimmed my admiration for him, not only as a teacher but as a human being. Of course, at that time I only knew him as a teacher, but he just made it all so clear and concise and scientific that it was a joy. So I would say those were the two major people who influenced my decision on St. Vincent's.

JGLP: You did make a career for yourself there. In fact, when you say Ed Hanin's name to anyone connected with St. Vincent's, at least among those to whom I've spoken, people smile. Really, a big smile comes to their faces. You are obviously someone who is very important and well-liked within that system.

DR. HANIN: You've talked to people about me? *[Laughs]*

JGLP: You already raised the issue of the difficulty of just being a psychiatrist in a Catholic hospital in the 1950s. Do you have any thoughts on what it was like being a gay psychiatrist working in a Catholic hospital throughout your career?

DR. HANIN: Yes. I think that the way I handled it was as much a rationalization as a reality. Looking back on it, I felt that as a person with a significant position in a Catholic institution, that I would not be active or vigorous in terms of proclaiming my gayness. Now this did not mean that I would pretend to be what I wasn't—

because I never did that. But I did feel that "the deal," in essence, was that I could do whatever I wanted to do in my private life, as long as I wasn't identified as gay in terms of my professional career. I say I think it's more of a rationalization than a reality because I'm not sure if I had been more vigorous or active, if it would have made a bit of difference. I know others have worked within the system very, very differently. But that, at least at that point in my life, was the way in which I dealt with it until my retirement from St. Vincent's. I never pretended to be what I wasn't. I never acted in ways that were different, but at the same time I was not very vocal within the gay psychiatric community.

JGLP: How did being gay affect you during training?

DR. HANIN: I think being gay really affected me in other, much more significant ways. For example, when I was in training, certainly a major part of the career path of a psychiatrist, especially one who was going to be involved in academic activities, was analytic training. I knew that there was no way that I could go into analytic training without leaving out a whole portion of my life, which made no sense to me. If I brought it up, that would certainly end my connection with the analytic institute. I always made the joke that I was a poor struggling student—in those days we didn't earn very much as house staff—and that I had a choice of either going into analytic training or getting a subscription to the Metropolitan Opera. So I chose the opera! And there is a kernel of truth to that. But, of course, the real reason I didn't pursue analytic training was that I knew that was not a way that I could comfortably go. So in that respect, being gay certainly did have a significant impact. I'm not sure that psychoanalysis was the career I would have decided upon anyway, but being gay was a major factor in how I proceeded in the areas of psychiatry into which I went.

JGLP: Could you talk about your personal relationship?

DR. HANIN: Well, I've been in a relationship with someone for more than forty-seven years. It began just before I entered medical school. It's a very important relationship to me, and he really has been very supportive and sustaining. People gasp in amazement that two men could be together for forty-seven years. Well, first, you have to be old. That helps. Then it takes a certain amount of apathy to keep the thing going on. But obviously a relationship takes work. I can't say it's always been smooth, but for the most part—

on the part of both of us—you work at it. And that's made it possible. It's obviously one of the most important things in my life, if not the most important. What else would you want to know about it? *[Laughs]*

JGLP: You mentioned that you were able to bring him into your professional life.

DR. HANIN: It was never an issue. People just basically accepted it, in the same way that someone else could bring a wife or a partner. That was just it; it was expected. That was in the APA. In terms of the hospital, no. That I wouldn't do. That would seem to me to cross a line that I didn't feel was right to cross. But on the other hand, I wouldn't take a woman date to the balls either. I would come just on my own. But certainly in terms of the APA, where I didn't feel that kind of "don't ask, don't tell" agreement, as it were, it was simply never an issue. And people could not have been more welcoming. And again, I say, I have a feeling that the way I handled things at work had a lot more to do with me than it necessarily had to do with the system. I certainly don't want to imply that the system would not have been accepting, but that was just the way I wanted to do it. You know, people think there was no gay life before Stonewall. But there was. There were places that you went and there was a large circle of friends that we had. New York City was someplace where one could be gay, and it didn't really make that much of a difference. I'm not sure I could have said the same thing if my career was someplace else, but certainly in New York City it was simply not an issue.

JGLP: You have played a very important part, and continue to play an important part, in the governance of the American Psychiatric Association. Could you talk about your APA involvement, past and present?

DR. HANIN: Well, as I said, in 1973, I went up to the Westchester branch of St. Vincent's in Harrison and became involved in the Westchester Psychiatric Association. Although I continued to live in New York City, I did feel that my professional life was going to be in Westchester. My involvement there was really the only way to make the hospital prominent in the Westchester area, to develop the kinds of networking that one needed to do. So I immediately joined the Westchester District Branch and proceeded to become involved there, eventually becoming president of that district branch in the late 1970s. Westchester had a tradition of moving their past presidents to the APA Assembly. So I became one of the two representatives from the Westchester branch to the assembly. Through the assembly elections, I became the recorder, and eventually the speaker of the assembly in 1991.

JGLP: You were an assembly representative when the gay caucus, and other minority caucuses, were given an assembly vote. How did that process unfold?

DR. HANIN: At that time, the whole issue of minorities in the assembly was a very controversial one. When the minority caucuses were first brought into the assembly—the black psychiatrists, the Asian Americans, the Hispanics, women, and the Native Americans and Pacific Islanders—it was basically with a token vote. Part of the deal was that every three years or so, on a rotating basis, they had to present a document showing why they should continue in the assembly—basically, to demonstrate that they represented an underserved population which was discriminated against, and which needed representation in the assembly. However, the idea of voting minority caucuses went against the whole way in which the APA Assembly had been developed and organized. Originally, it had been an assembly of district branches. In any event, it was just a token. If the assembly were to vote by strength, for example, the New York County District Branch has about 2,000 votes. Yet, each minority group had only one. So they were hardly going to overturn the assembly, even though they did provide a voice for minority issues within the assembly. Nevertheless, there was a real reluctance to go beyond the initial group of minorities.

JGLP: Meaning ethnic minorities?

DR. HANIN: Ethnic minorities and women as a minority. Eventually, two new groups sought acknowledgment as minorities. One was the Caucus of Gay, Lesbian, and Bisexual Psychiatrists, and later the International Medical Graduates (IMGs). It's not that people in the assembly were not open to some of the issues that gay psychiatrists were bringing up. After all, there were already within the APA a group of psychiatrists who were clearly identifying themselves as gay, as opposed to sort of sliding under the radar, as it were. It wasn't that people were opposed to the idea of a vote for the GLB caucus; it's that people didn't quite know how to deal with it. They didn't quite know how to fit this type of representation into a governing body that had developed as representing individual district branches. So there was a very, very lively debate in the assembly. But it did pass there and was then passed by the board of trustees. So now we had, among the minority groups, an established gay entity that could speak to the issues, not just for psychiatrists who were gay, but, more important, for patients who were gay. That was really their role. Of course that became very significant, particularly in terms of other, later developments that occurred over the years when American psychiatry became much more comfortable with the issue of gayness, and sexuality in general, than it was when I first came to the assembly.

At some point I chaired the Committee on Planning of the APA Assembly, and one thing we did of which I am frankly proudest is getting rid of the need for minority groups to constantly justify their presence in the assembly. So much effort went into developing documents to justify their continuing in the assembly, rather than pushing forward the needs of their constituency and the patient groups for which they were advocating. So at least we got that out of the way. One of the things upon which I was very clear when I decided to run for office in the assembly, first as recorder, and then as speaker-elect, and—I guess even before that as area rep—is that I was not going to come in under any false colors. I made very sure at that particular point in time that my partner was very much a presence. I didn't go to executive committee dinners alone. I didn't want to make a big deal about it, but if I was going to run for office, I wanted people to know who I was.

JGLP: And that worked?

DR. HANIN: It worked. Again, on a personal level, I developed very good friendships within the APA. People have been really very accepting. It's simply not an issue for a lot of people when you're talking about a personal relationship. It's very different when you're talking about being gay in broader terms, and other issues begin to come into it.

After my term as speaker, I was asked to chair the Joint Commission on Public Affairs, which I did for three years. I eventually ran for vice president of APA in 1993, but I lost the election. However, I don't think my being gay had anything to do with that. I just didn't run a very good campaign—and I discovered I really didn't like campaigning.

Within the assembly—I guess it was like Congress in a way—you dealt with relatively small groups, and you could do a fair amount of things behind the scenes. Running for office in the APA really meant vigorously campaigning to the entire membership, and it's just not something with which I was comfortable. So I took the defeat as instruction from above that I shouldn't do this again—and I didn't. But I continued to be active in the APA. I chaired the Council on National Affairs, which is actually the council to which all of the minority committees report. I already mentioned the Joint Commission on Public Affairs—I was on a number of panels of that sort, commissions, ad hoc task forces, various things. And certainly in more recent years I have reduced my level of activity within the APA. It's time for the younger members to come up and do it. And I can't think of anything worse than people who can't let go and, you know, really feel they have to hang on for dear life.

JGLP: Although you were not in a position of authority within APA governance in 1973 when the APA removed homosexuality from the *Diagnostic and Statistical Manual,* you were a member of the APA. What do you remember about that time and how did you experience it?

DR. HANIN: I remember a couple of things. One, it was very controversial, and the controversy was led by people who essentially said that this was politics intruding into science. It wasn't. The APA Board of Trustees had reviewed very carefully the evidence related to homosexuality. A lot of that evidence was brought to them by the group of psychiatrists who were willing to identify themselves as gay and to advocate for this change. I do remember being at the 1970 plenary session in San Francisco that was disrupted by protesters to bring the issue to the attention of psychiatrists. Many psychiatrists then, and maybe even today, clearly felt that homosexuality and heterosexuality were not equal. Certainly at that time, most, if not all of us, were trained that homosexuality was, if not an illness, then a distortion of psychosexual development which resulted from troubled relationships with domineering, seductive mothers and absent fathers. You know, the whole schmeer—that was what was taught. This was not a fringe group saying this. This was American psychiatry. And of course they said that the goal of psychiatry should be to "cure" homosexuality.

So deleting homosexuality took psychiatry in a different direction. It met with a lot of opposition, especially from those groups who were analytically oriented. And they actually got a petition to challenge this by calling for a referendum of the membership—who, fortunately, supported the actions of the board.[1] But at that time, this was not an easy idea, I think, for a lot of psychiatrists to accept in practice. It was a fairly radical step, in many ways far more radical than the later removal of ego-dystonic homosexuality from the nomenclature.[2] The 1973 decision really made everything that followed possible. First, it was a rather brave step on the part of the American Psychiatric Association, and for American psychiatry. Unlike some later moves, where other groups were far in advance of the APA, like reparative therapy and same-sex unions, here American psychiatry showed it could lead. Second, this action showed that American psychiatry could admit an error; that what it had been essentially teaching and training—what had been, in a sense, part of the warp and woof of analytic thinking—was not so. That, I think, took a lot of courage. It would have been a lot easier to push everything away. It was an exciting time in a lot of ways and, I think, made a tremendous difference.

JGLP: Did the change have any personal meaning to you as a gay psychiatrist in 1973?

DR. HANIN: I remember that for a number of years prior to 1973, the gay psychiatrists would meet clandestinely during the APA, hidden away from others, and not part of the official program. After 1973 it was out in the open. Now this did not change the way in which I operated, what I did in any of my roles, either in my hospital career or in the APA. That part didn't change. But there was a different feel.

I must add that one of the things I've been most content with, in terms of my involvement with APA, has been on the Council on National Affairs. I think it's the place where I've been most helpful because, as I said, I was not really involved in the early battles. I've never been a member of the GLB Caucus, although I am a member of AGLP. My activity in psychiatry has really been away from the whole issue. However, I think I was helpful in the whole area of moving the APA to take a position on reparative therapy. I'm pleased I was able to help with that. The initiative has been stalled for many years. As I learned from Dr. Tompkins, people sometimes have the idea that if they are right, and if they make the argument strong enough, that others are just going to say, "Sure, yes." But life just doesn't work that way. It's important to know how to move an idea through a complex governance structure to be able to achieve what one wants to achieve. It's not that people don't want to go along with you; it's just that one has to marshal arguments and to go through a certain process. It's like getting a bill through Congress. It really is—like campaign finance reform or whatever. I believe I was helpful in guiding those who developed the policy and statements on reparative therapy, to show them how to move it along. I'm very pleased with that. I really am.

JGLP: I know you are enjoying many aspects of your retirement. As you said, you didn't go into psychoanalysis but went to the opera instead. Could you talk about your work at the Metropolitan Opera.

DR. HANIN: Well, in the August—or is it the fall?—of my life, I have started a new career doing backstage tours at the Metropolitan Opera. I find it a lot of fun. Now I have not disappeared from psychiatry entirely. I still do some teaching at the hospital. I teach the course on ethics in psychiatry, and a course on dynamic formulation. However, at least once a week. I'm at the opera house taking groups of people around the backstage. I'm showing them things and learning an awful lot at the same time. The opera is something of which I've always been very, very fond. I really did get a subscription way back when I was a resident. That was not a story. Now I don't sit quite so high in the bleachers as I did when I was younger. I also don't stand at the opera anymore, as I used to. It's kind of fun.

JGLP: Is there anything else you might want to tell us?

DR. HANIN: No, I think you've really covered my life quite succinctly. You know, it's not the most exciting one. But it's a fairly comfortable one. It's most interesting for me to see the shifts in attitudes that have occurred in my lifetime, not only in society in general, but also within the profession. I think that there is an acceptance, but that acceptance is not per se equality. I'm talking now, not only of society in general, but even within our field. I think we are seeing a certain amount of political correctness, but not necessarily a heartfelt acceptance of equality, at least in terms of lifestyle or partner of choice. But we are so far from where we were, that we haven't achieved nirvana seems not such a bad thing. It at least gives us something to work toward.

NOTES

1. Editor's Note: For a detailed chronicle of these events, see Bayer, R. (1981), *Homosexuality and American Psychiatry: The Politics of Diagnosis*. New York: Basic Books.

2. Editor's Note: For an account of that development, see Krajeski, J. (1996), Homosexuality and the mental health professions. In: *Textbook of Homosexuality and Mental Health,* ed. R. Cabaj & T. Stein. Washington, DC: American Psychiatric Press, pp. 17-31.

Chapter 17

An Interview with Ralph E. Roughton, MD

Paul E. Lynch

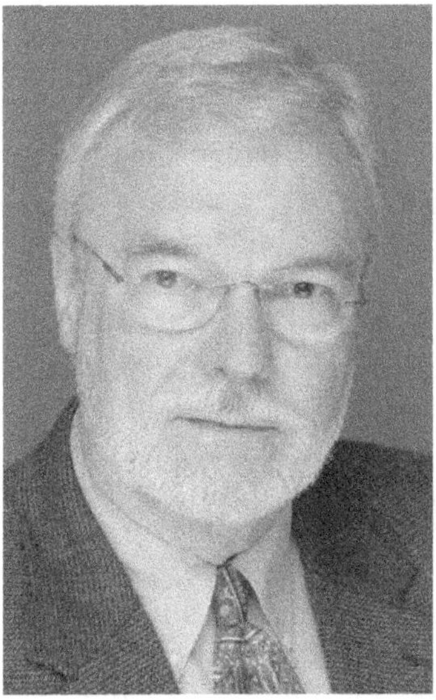

Ralph Roughton, MD, is Training and Supervising Psychoanalyst at the Emory University Psychoanalytic Institute, where he served as Education Director from 1983-1986, and Director of the Institute from 1986-1991. He is also Clinical Professor in the Emory University Department of Psychiatry and Behavioral Sciences.

In 1991, Dr. Roughton was appointed the first Chair of the American Psychoanalytic Association's (APsaA) Committee on Issues of Homosexuality (currently known as the Committee on Gay and Lesbian Issues). In this role, Dr. Roughton's goal was to disseminate and implement the APsaA's newly created policy of nondiscrimination against gay and lesbian candidates—a policy that had been adopted by the APsaA in 1991 after years of contentious debate. He spoke at psychoanalytic institutes across the United States, acted as a consultant to the institutes, and spoke frequently and frankly at the

This chapter appeared originally under the same title in *Journal of Gay & Lesbian Psychotherapy* 10(2):105-116.

American Psychiatry and Homosexuality: An Oral History

doi:10.1300/6049_18

meetings of the APsaA. In doing so, Dr. Roughton helped broaden and personalize discussions of homosexuality among American psychoanalysts. By 1999, when Dr. Roughton brought the proposition of a nondiscrimination policy to the International Psychoanalytic Association (IPA), he had the solid backing of American psychoanalysts, most of whom by that time considered Dr. Roughton a friend and respected colleague.

When he came out of the closet within the psychoanalytic profession in 1996, Dr. Roughton became the first openly gay training and supervising psychoanalyst to be recognized within the American and International Psychoanalytic Associations. He is a tireless supervisor, teacher, and consultant, and he sits on the editorial boards of several psychoanalytic journals. To acknowledge his achievements, the APsaA now offers an annual Ralph Roughton Award for Outstanding Contributions to the Literature on Homosexuality in his honor.

JGLP: Your accent gives away your roots in the American South, and here you are, a late bloomer, but a gay activist nonetheless. How and where did your journey begin?

DR. ROUGHTON: In a small town, Sandersville, in middle Georgia. My father was a businessman, who ran a grocery store, then a furniture shop. My mother taught piano in our home. My father was also mayor of the town, a part-time job for which I doubt he even got paid. But during World War II, we did receive a slightly bigger ration of gasoline because he was the mayor. He was also something of an athlete. He played semiprofessional baseball until he was in his forties, and then he took up golf and became a local champ. Eventually my brother-in-law and sister took over the furniture store. I remain close to them, and they continue to live in the town where we grew up.

JGLP: Where did you go to college and medical school, and what was it like for you away from Sandersville?

DR. ROUGHTON: I went to Duke University for both college (1950-1953) and medical school (1953-1957). I wanted to go north to school, but North Carolina was as far as I could get. Still, it was an eye-opening experience. I had grown up in a very religious family—Southern Methodist—where everything was seen as either right or wrong. I was a product of that environment and had to get beyond it. Being from a small town in the deep South, Duke and the people I met there broadened my experience. The Methodist student group was more liberal than our home church, and then I eventually found my way to the Unitarian church. My other main college activity was working on the Duke yearbook as assistant editor.

My first choice for medical school was Duke. I liked the people and knew others who would be going there. The main thing that comes to mind about medical school is how uptight I was. I was always eager to please and kept my nose to the grindstone. I had always been in a hurry to get through school—I finished college in three years. Medical school was pretty much the same—a lot of work and not much play.

I got married during my second year, and we became part of the more serious group of married students. My wife had also grown up in the same small town—in fact, our grandparents had been neighbors, and our families were lifelong friends. That's rare today, but not so unusual in that time and place.

JGLP: What was life like after medical school, and what led you to psychiatry and psychoanalysis?

DR. ROUGHTON: I first became interested in psychiatry during high school, when I saw the movie *The Snake Pit.* I wanted to be the handsome doctor who cured Olivia de Havilland. It was not until years later that I realized it was my mother I was hoping to cure, rather than Olivia. But in medical school, I thought the psychiatrists I met were all weird people, and I did not want to become weird; so I decided I would be a general practitioner instead. Also, my maternal grandfather was a horse-and-buggy doctor, and I suppose that had some influence on me.

I came to Atlanta for a two-year general practice residency at Grady Memorial Hospital (1957-1959), and our first daughter was born here during my internship. Then I owed the air force three years, and they sent me to Japan in 1959, where I was a general medical officer taking care of the servicemen and their dependents. Our second daughter was born in Japan. We liked Japan but didn't get to travel much because the children were small. Our interest in Japanese culture, however, led us to choose a contemporary Japanese-style house when we came back to Atlanta. After three years as a medical officer, my interest in psychiatry had revived, and I came to Emory for a psychiatry residency in 1962. There was a strong psychoanalytic emphasis in the department, and I continued with that, graduating from the Emory Psychoanalytic Institute in 1972.

JGLP: I know that you have an interest and some academic background in literature. Did you pursue any other interests, and how did your avocational interests fit in with medical and psychiatric obligations?

DR. ROUGHTON: I rushed through college as a premed, so I had no time for anything else then. At a time when the Emory Institute appeared to be on shaky ground trying to get established, I went back to school to study literature. I was working on a master's degree, and then the institute turned around. I was appointed education director, and from that point the institute pretty much took up all of my time, so I never finished the master's degree.

My other great interest was music. My mother was a piano teacher and started me with lessons at age four. In my last two years of high school, I studied with a teacher at a nearby conservatory, and I won a statewide competition. I also sang in the Atlanta Symphony Chorus with Robert Shaw and performed in some U.S. tours, including several Carnegie Hall performances. I am playing the piano again, now that institute work has slowed some for me. Now I am trying to get back to the level I was playing in high school—even working on pieces I played in the contest.

JGLP: You certainly have earned a little playtime, although you have not yet retired. You have worked hard on the national level and been instrumental in the sea change in the American Psychoanalytic Association with regard to homosexuality.

DR. ROUGHTON: I've been around to see more changes than I ever thought possible.

JGLP: Prior to the changes in psychoanalysis, 1973 was a big year for many gay psychiatrists because the American Psychiatric Association (APA) removed homosexuality from its list of mental disorders. What were you doing at the time, and did the APA decision have any immediate impact on your professional or personal life?

DR. ROUGHTON: I had finished my psychoanalytic training the year before, in 1972, and I was not active in the APA. I am not sure when I became aware of the APA decision. I did not attend APA meetings—except when they were in Atlanta—until a few years ago, when I went to an AGLP [Association of Gay and Lesbian Psychiatrists] meeting to talk about the recent changes toward gay people in the APsaA.

In 1972, I was working as a psychiatrist and psychoanalyst, married and raising children. Everything I did professionally, I did as a heterosexual psychiatrist. I was heterosexual as far as the world could see. I still felt that it would be better to overcome my homosexual feelings. That same year, I started my second analysis, again trying to get rid of homosexual feelings after a first analysis had failed to accomplish that.

From today's perspective, that was such a tragic mistake and so harmful. But in the 1970s, that is what we did. We tried to become straight, and our analysts told us we could.

I attended my first APsaA meeting in 1976, and it just happened that at that meeting there was a panel on "The Psychoanalytic Treatment of Male Homosexuality," with Robert Stoller, Ethel Person, and Charles Socarides.[1] All three spoke about the etiology, defining the pathology, and talking about treatment. Of course, Stoller and Person went on to make major changes in their views; Socarides did not.

A more significant moment for me, though, was in 1984, when Dick Isay organized a panel with himself, Stan Leavy, Rick Friedman, and Stoller, again—but with a very different message this time. Now we heard for the first time that homosexuality was not a priori pathological. This represented a major shift, largely due to Dick Isay's efforts as chair of the program committee, even though he was not himself out of the closet at that point.

To get back to your question about the 1973 APA decision—had I known, my take on it would have been, "Okay. It's good to know that we're not crazy." Certainly the APA decision is one of many things that contributed over the next twenty years to my coming out professionally in 1996. At that time, I was up for reappointment as a training analyst at the Emory Psychoanalytic Institute, and I wanted to know that my colleagues were making the decision to reappoint me, or not, with full knowledge of who I am.

JGLP: You became a training analyst in 1979. Did you worry about your homosexuality affecting that appointment?

DR. ROUGHTON: Oh, yes. I was always quite anxious about exposure—always self-conscious about mannerisms and watching what I said—always hoping not to give myself away. It was the climate of the times. It was not long after the time of McCarthyism, and there were actually more homosexuals hounded out of government jobs by those witch hunts than Communists. It was also around the time that Howard Brown resigned as the New York City Health Commissioner in order to avoid being outed—it was only later that he came out and wrote his book.[2] There was a terrible climate of fear because being exposed as a homosexual meant being ruined.

JGLP: Despite these fears, you continued to advance in the psychoanalytic world.

DR. ROUGHTON: Yes, I was involved in committee work of both the Emory Psychoanalytic Institute and the APsaA, starting in the mid-1970s, and remain active today. I have also taught a good deal at the Emory Institute. I became the education director for the Emory Psychoanalytic Institute in 1983, and the director of the institute in 1986. Then I felt even more pressure and constraint because, as my positions were more prominent, I knew any exposure of me also meant scandal for the institute. At the time Emory was a new and developing institute, under the wings of the Columbia Institute, and I feared that exposure of the institute's director as a "homosexual" would discredit the entire institute.

JGLP: During these decades that you were closeted, the world was changing. Laws were changing, and gay and lesbian people were becoming more and more visible. Were you paying attention to what was going on outside the psychoanalytic world?

DR. ROUGHTON: Yes, I was paying attention. But I was also still married, and the father of two children. I thought about whether it would be possible to be an "out" gay analyst and what that would be like. But thoughts about my personal life and what was going on in my marriage were the overriding concerns. I might have come out sooner and been more of a pioneer, if I had been more comfortable with myself as a gay man. And, of course, the focus in my personal analysis had been on trying to change my sexual feelings, not accept them, and that was no help.

JGLP: Yet you did get involved with gay issues in the APsaA before you came out. How did that happen?

DR. ROUGHTON: I got involved in 1991, at the time of APsaA's passage of a resolution barring discrimination on the basis of homosexuality. I was on the APsaA's Executive Council at the time, and of course voted for the resolution—although I had not been actively involved in the process of getting it passed. Then there was an article in the APsaA's newsletter, *The American Psychoanalyst (TAP),* by Joanna Chapin, in which she interviewed both Isay and Socarides. The article made it clear to me that it was going to be a long time before this new nondiscrimination policy was widely accepted by the membership.

I wrote a letter to the chair of the Board on Professional Standards (BOPS) and the editor of *TAP,* suggesting that the passing of the policy needed to be followed up by a committee to oversee implementation of the policy. At the time, Bernard Pacella was president of APsaA and Marvin Margolis was chair of the BOPS, and they decided to form a joint committee (of BOPS and the executive council), and they asked me to chair it. Once the nondiscrimination policy was passed, I saw a different attitude from the leaders of APsaA. There was a gradually increasing awareness of the changes that were coming.

The following year, in May 1992, there was a vote to add wording to specifically state that progression to training and supervising analyst is also covered by the nondiscrimination policy. It was the fall of 1992 when the Committee on Homosexual Issues was formed, and we had our first meeting during the December meetings of that year.

JGLP: At that time, the only openly gay analyst in the APsaA was Richard Isay, and he was not on the committee. How did you recruit the other members of the committee, and why was Isay not on it?

DR. ROUGHTON: Dick Isay deserves a lot of credit for the changes in the APsaA.[3] He broke down the doors, and then others among us came in to work in a more collaborative way. I discussed the committee with Dick as it was being formed, and we discussed the fact that he had become "political poison." He was very angry, for many good reasons, but he had become a lightning rod for contention. He had burned too many bridges. It did not seem to me that his presence on the committee would advance our goals of identifying and ending discrimination and broadening discussion of the issues of homosexuality. Dick's aggressive approach had been necessary to force change in the APsaA, but it was not my style and not what I felt was needed at that time to help people accept the changes. My maxim was always, "When people begin moving in the right direction, stop kicking them."

I do not recall how each of the other members came to my attention, but in one way or another each of them had indicated an interest in homosexual issues. The initial members included three former directors of institutes and the president-elect of the APsaA, so it was a group with some clout in the organization. I invited Houston MacIntosh because he had done a survey of analysts' attitudes on homosexuality,[4] and his preliminary reports of this seemed reasonable. It turned out that he was more interested in defending analysts against charges of homophobia than he was in implementing the nondiscrimination policy. So we came to a joint decision that this committee was not the place for him.

JGLP: Can you say a little about the highlights of the committee work, and the events that most significantly shifted attitudes within APsaA?

DR. ROUGHTON: Well, the first would have to be the battle that Socarides and his group fought even after the nondiscrimination policy was approved. They threatened a legal challenge and wanted a referendum. There were many meetings where I would get up and speak counter to Socarides, and I became more and more confident of my position and answers as this continued. Also a great deal of this played out in print in *TAP.*

A significant turning point was when *TAP* ran an advertisement for Socarides' group, the National Association for Research and Therapy of Homosexuality (NARTH). Bill Jeffries, the editor of *TAP,* and others were treating it as a controversy with two sides that deserved equal print space and failed to see that we were an official committee of the association. After a lot of commotion, a few of us—you included, Paul—were invited to meet with the executive committee. I think that meeting was a real turning point because it caused the executive committee to come out very publicly, with a written statement in *TAP,* giving their full backing to the work of our committee.

I think the 1998 public forum "Homophobia: Analysis of a Permissible Prejudice," which you chaired, Paul, was also a highlight.[5] That was a wonderful collaboration of the Committee on Public Information and the Committee on Issues of Homosexuality to educate the APsaA membership and the interested public. I think it showed that APsaA was taking a new stance. We had been part of the problem of homophobia, and now we were becoming part of the solution.

After that, things happened quickly. When you suggested that APsaA endorse a resolution in favor of gay marriage from Lambda Legal Defense, I was surprised by how readily it was taken up and approved, almost unanimously, with only one question raised about use of the word "marriage." Then, of course, other resolutions followed, in favor of gay adoption and parenting, and against treatments geared to changing sexual orientation.

JGLP: In your usual manner, you did not mention the plenary address that you were invited to give at the 2001 meeting of APsaA. Your invitation was certainly a sign of the change that had taken place, and your plenary speech to the membership of APsaA, another major contribution to the education and change of the association.

DR. ROUGHTON: Well, that is true—for me personally, the plenary was the highlight of my career. It was also special for me that my daughters came to New Orleans to be in the audience, and to celebrate the occasion. I was also happy that it happened to be the tenth anniversary—almost to the day—of the nondiscrimination policy's passage, although the program committee had not been aware of that when they invited me to give the plenary address. But that made looking back on the ten years of change the obvious topic for my address.

JGLP: What effect did those years of committee work have on you personally?

DR. ROUGHTON: I certainly became more and more politically identified with the issue (of homosexuality), and it sort of allowed me to try on the identity. Working with Susan Vaughan, Sidney Phillips, and you, Paul, gave me the opportunity to form personal relationships with gay people, and also to see that it was possible to have a professional life and be a gay analyst. All this was happening in parallel with what was going on in my personal life. I was still married when I was invited to chair the committee, and my wife and I discussed the invitation. I was willing to take the risk, and although she was reluctant and frightened about what it might mean for our marriage and our family for me to become publicly identified with the controversy over homosexuality, she was supportive. My wife and I separated later, in the summer of 1993.

JGLP: Prior to the 1998 panel on homophobia, you agreed to be interviewed by Erica Goode, and photographed, for an article that ran in the *New York Times.*[6] Once you were out, you did not hold back at all. Were there any particular events that helped you, or forced you, to come out?

DR. ROUGHTON: I don't think so. The committee and the people I worked with were one influence, but it happened gradually over a period of several years. It was a process that was mostly internal—coming to terms with my sexuality and with my marriage—that went along in parallel with my professional considerations.

There was one event in the fall of 1994 where I considered coming out, two years before I actually did. The Columbia Psychoanalytic Center was having a faculty retreat to discuss newer thinking about homosexuality, and they invited me to give a paper on bisexuality. At the time, I had already separated from my wife, I had been chair of the Committee on Issues of Homosexuality for two years, and I was becoming increasingly identified with the subject. I considered revealing my sexual orientation as part of that presentation. I discussed it with Rick Friedman, who was a member of the Columbia faculty and a friend, and he advised me not to do it. He felt that many of the faculty would discredit what I had to say if it came from a gay man. He may have been right for that time in an institute with a notorious history of antihomosexual statements from many of its former members (Rado, Kardiner, Socarides, as well as my own training analyst). We will never know the answer, but two years later when I did come out professionally, the reception could not have been more personally warm and accepting.

JGLP: In 1997, we were both in Barcelona for the meetings of the International Psychoanalytic Association (IPA). You were speaking on a panel about homosexuality,[7] and the brief description of the panel in the program began with a question like, "Homosexuality—What kind of pathology is it?" I was very proud when you identified yourself as a gay training analyst to that hostile audience, particularly as your presentation was juxtaposed with the pathologizing views presented by the French and South American analysts on the panel. Was that the first time you identified yourself publicly as a gay analyst, and was that a difficult decision to make?

DR. ROUGHTON: I had come out professionally in 1996 by writing letters to all of my local colleagues, to analysts I knew at Columbia, and to significant people I knew in the APsaA, including the officers who had appointed me to the committee. So I was publicly out, but I had not yet stood up before an audience and said, "I am gay."

But at that panel in Barcelona, I was dealing with more than whether or not to come out because I was recuperating from coronary angioplasty. I had actually delayed going to the doctor about my chest pains for several weeks, partly because I was afraid I would have to have bypass surgery and miss the trip to Barcelona. It turned out that all I needed was angioplasty and a stent, so I had that done just three weeks before standing up on that stage and declaring myself a gay training analyst. I was still taking anticoagulants and a bit shaky from the anaphylactic reaction I had during the angioplasty. However, I forgot about that when the panel moderator first began his introduction by quoting Socarides, and then the analyst from Argentina presented her psychotic patient as "a case of homosexuality," and finally the first comment from the audience linked homosexuals and pedophiles. Thinking back to that moment, it is not surprising that it took another five years to get the IPA to adopt a nondiscrimination policy.

JGLP: In addition to that brave panel presentation, you also worked politically for change in the IPA. Can you say a little about that?

DR. ROUGHTON: I was elected by the executive council to represent APsaA in the IPA House of Delegates. I had made it known that if elected to be the representative, I would introduce a nondiscrimination policy similar to what we now had in APsaA.

In Santiago, Chile, in 1999, the house of delegates passed the nondiscrimination policy that I proposed, but the IPA Executive Council took out all reference to homosexuality before they passed it. So what we got was a very bland, nonspecific policy of nondiscrimination. There was a big backlash, primarily from American analysts, and the house of delegates asked the executive council to reconsider. In Nice, France, in 2001, the executive council again rejected any of the wording that specified that homosexuals were not to be discriminated against. This time there was an even bigger backlash, spreading to the APsaA membership on the "openline" e-mail discussion group.

I was joined by the APsaA's Executive Council in writing to the president of IPA, Professor Widlocher, asking if the general statement of nondiscrimination includes homosexuality. In this way we forced them to answer. The answer that came back was, "Yes, it did include homosexuality." Widlocher then asked the (small) IPA Executive Committee to present the policy to the (larger) IPA Executive Council as their own motion, and they did. After another heated debate, the executive council did pass language similar to our original proposal.[8]

JGLP: After all of these heated debates, politicking, and scientific presentations, have you any suggestions for others who would work to change antigay feelings and policies?

DR. ROUGHTON: Knowing people as individuals is the key to overcoming prejudice. Creating a climate that allows people to come out and let others get to know them is invaluable to changing people's feelings. When I came out in a letter to my colleagues at the Emory Institute and to the Executive Committee of APsaA, Marvin Margolis was the president of APsaA. He said to me, "Ralph, this isn't going to change the way people feel about you. It is going to change the way people think about homosexuality." I think that encapsulates what my role has been in the process of change in American Psychoanalysis.

NOTES

1. Wiedeman, G.H. & Payne, E.C. (1977), The psychoanalytic treatment of male homosexuality. *J. Amer. Psychoanal. Assn.,* 25:183-199.

2. Brown, H. (1976), *Familiar Faces, Hidden Lives: The Story of Homosexual Men in America Today.* New York: Harcourt, Brace Jovanovich.

3. Isay, R. (1996), *Becoming Gay: The Journey to Self-Acceptance.* New York: Pantheon.

4. MacIntosh, H. (1994), Attitudes and experiences of psychoanalysts in analyzing homosexual patients. *J. Amer. Psychoanal. Assn.,* 42:1183-1207.

5. Hoffman, L.G., Hevesi, A.G., Lynch, P.E., Gomes, P.J., Chodorow, N.J., Roughton, R.E., Frank, B. & Vaughan, S. (2000), Homophobia: Analysis of a "permissible prejudice." *J. Gay & Lesbian Psychother.,* 4(1):5-53.

6. Goode, E. (1998), On gay issues, psychoanalysis treats itself. *The New York Times* (Arts & Ideas Section), December 12, pp. A19, A29.

7. Berman, E. (1998), Homosexuality. *Int. J. Psycho-Anal.,* 79:806-810.

8. Roughton, R. (2003), The International Psychoanalytical Association and homosexuality. *J. Gay & Lesbian Psychotherapy,* 7(1/2):189-196. Reprinted in: *The Mental Health Professions and Homosexuality: International Perspectives,* ed. V. Lingiardi & J. Drescher. Binghamton, NY: The Haworth Press, pp. 189-196.

SELECTED BIBLIOGRAPHY

Roughton, R. (2000), Homophobia and the American Psychoanalytic Association. In: Homophobia: Analysis of a "permissible" prejudice. A public forum of the American Psychoanalytic Association and the American Psychoanalytic Foundation. *J. Gay & Lesbian Psychotherapy,* 4(1):28-35.

Roughton, R. (2000), Sometimes a desire is just a desire: A response to Jack Drescher's "Psychoanalytic Therapy and the Gay Man," *Gender & Psychoanalysis,* 5:259-273.

Roughton, R. (2001), Four men in treatment: An evolving perspective on homosexuality and bisexuality, 1965-2000. *J. American Psychoanalytic Association,* 49: 1187-1217.

Roughton, R. (2001), Homosexuality: Clinical and technical issues. *International Psychoanalysis,* 10(1):17-19.

Roughton, R. (2001), Dialogue on homosexuality—Continued. *International Psychoanalysis,* 10(2):29-32.

Roughton, R. (2002), Being gay and becoming a psychoanalyst: Across three generations. *J. Gay & Lesbian Psychotherapy,* 6(1):31-43.

Roughton, R. (2002), Opportunities missed [essay in memory of Stephen Mitchell]. *Studies in Gender & Sexuality,* 3:73-82.

Roughton, R. (2002), Response to Bergeret's "Homosexuality or homoeroticism: 'Narcissistic eroticism'." *International J. Psycho-analysis,* 83:949-953.

Roughton, R. (2002), Rethinking homosexuality: What it teaches us about psychoanalysis. Plenary address. *J. American Psychoanalytic Association,* 50:733-763.

Roughton, R. (2002), The two analyses of a gay man: The interplay between social change and psychoanalytic understanding. *Annual of Psychoanalysis,* 30:83-99.

Roughton, R. (2003), The International Psychoanalytical Association and homosexuality. *J. Gay & Lesbian Psychotherapy,* 7(1/2):189-196. Reprinted in: *The Mental Health Professions and Homosexuality: International Perspectives,* ed. V. Lingiardi & J. Drescher. Binghamton, NY: The Haworth Press, pp. 189-196.

Afterword: Today and Tomorrow

Mary E. Barber

We have come a long way in a short time. In 1972, a masked John Fryer feared for his career as he spoke about being a gay psychiatrist. Thirty-three years later, Jack Drescher, openly gay psychiatrist and author of a major body of work on gay-affirmative therapy (Drescher, 1998), is nominated to run for president of the American Psychiatric Association (APA) (Melzer, 2005) and Joseph P. Merlino was named the first openly gay psychoanalyst to serve as president of a national medical psychoanalytic group, the American Academy of Psychoanalysis and Dynamic Psychiatry (2004-2006). Not long ago there was little, if any, popular media representation of gay people. And when there was, as in *The Boys in the Band,* homosexuality was portrayed in tragic terms. We now have *Will and Grace, Queer Eye for the Straight Guy,* and Ellen Degeneres' current success as an openly gay comedian and talk show host. In the legal arena, we have seen the end of antisodomy laws and moves toward marriage equality in Massachusetts—not to mention Canada, Belgium, the Netherlands, South Africa, and Spain. We are truly at the dawn of a "queer millennium" (Rosario, 2002).

Ironically, our successes as gay mental health professionals have put us in the odd position of needing to justify our ongoing work. When the APA recently approved a position statement in support of same-sex civil marriages (APA, 2005), the main opposition to its passage came from members who argued that gay and lesbian issues are *not* a psychiatric matter—that is to say, that if homosexuality is not a mental illness, then psychiatry should have nothing to say about the "social issue" of gay rights. At the same time, the Association of Gay and Lesbian Psychiatrists (AGLP), an allied organization of the APA,

American Psychiatry and Homosexuality: An Oral History

doi:10.1300/6049_19

created and sustained through the hard work and risk-taking of many of the people profiled in this book, has had to contend with apathy based on some of the same assumptions. Dubious members wonder why, if gay psychiatrists no longer have to hide and if gay patients are no longer pathologized by mainstream psychiatry, do we need an AGLP?

Activist Frank Kameny, one of those involved in the original APA protests, lost his civil service position when it was discovered he was gay. True, this does not generally occur today. And psychiatry stopped its damaging practice of screening out homosexuals from service after homosexuality was removed from the *Diagnostic and Statistical Manual* (DSM). However, thirty years later, the military continues to discharge gays and lesbians from service through the "Don't ask, Don't tell" policy. One wonders how far we have progressed since the times when some bravely resisted military protocol that excluded gays (Geltman, 2002; Merlino, 2001, and in this volume).

Nor has psychiatry's unfortunate legacy of trying to "cure" homosexuals completely disappeared, although the purveyors of such "therapies" have moved out of the mental health mainstream. Today, in place of past, misguided efforts to change people from gay to straight through psychoanalysis, we now have damaging efforts to change people through faith (Shidlo, Schroeder, and Drescher, 2001; Drescher and Zucker, 2006). Social conservative faith groups sponsoring "ex-gay" ministries and promoting "reparative therapies" are often better organized and funded than most medical or mental health organizations. Parents and young adults targeted by these groups often do not see information from mainstream psychiatry that would counter the message these groups are marketing. At the same time, mainstream mental health practitioners often view ex-gay ministries as fringe groups undeserving of our concern. Furthermore, since these groups do not operate in the scientific realm, they are *not* subject to scientific or ethical standards when making claims of efficacy or promoting their "treatments." That is to say, they can overstate (and even lie) about their "successes" and minimize or even deny the harm that they do.

So there are still vestiges of past injustices to battle. Even if psychiatry has effectively rendered its opinion with the 1973 deletion of homosexuality, the field must continue to correct the mistakes of our past. Psychiatry still bears responsibility for educating the public and disseminating the facts. As psychiatrists and mental health practitioners, we also have an ethical obligation to address "treatments" that affect quality of care and access to care for LGBT people. And if such treatments are being promoted outside of mainstream mental health practice, we need to extend our efforts beyond mental health professional circles to inform the general public. We need to wake our straight (and gay) colleagues from their apathy or dissuade them from the belief that addressing these issues is someone else's responsibility. Now that we have come out of the shadows and have a voice, we need to make that voice heard.

We also have new challenges and opportunities as LGBT mental health professionals. The increasingly visible transgender and intersex communities are raising questions and concerns about diagnosis, stigma and discrimination, and standards of treatment. Each new decade of the HIV pandemic brings challenges to LGBT people as treatments advance, as people living with HIV live longer, and as newer generations must still be educated about safer sex (Merlino, 1997). The growing number of families with children headed by same-sex couples need us to meet their mental health needs and advocate for appropriate societal supports.

These and other issues too numerous to name *are* social issues. And medical issues. And mental health issues. We, as lesbian, gay, bisexual, and transgender psychiatrists, are uniquely positioned to address these topics which fall well within the biopsychosocial framework we use for assessing individuals, families, and communities. We are able to do research, education, and advocacy on issues like these because of our unique training, and because we are standing on the shoulders of the pioneers profiled in this book.

Not only are we able. We *must* carry out this work. Many of us who participated in this book, either as interviewers or subjects, found the experience of telling and hearing these stories to be powerful and moving. These men and women did remarkable things, some leading to sudden change and some to incremental change, but collectively all making enormous steps forward for psychiatry and mental health. Often these individuals did what they did while otherwise just trying to make a living, make a career, and do what we all do to progress through our lives. Yet they are all heroes, pioneers, and fathers, mothers, brothers, and sisters to many of us who are coming up now.

We may think of ourselves as pretty nonheroic, often just trying to survive and cope with the many external stressors placed on mental health professionals these days. Yet we must remember that, as psychiatrists and mental health professionals, we are in a place of privilege in our communities and that, as LGBT people, we are generally no longer in fear of our lives and jobs within our profession. We have grown comfortable with our newfound safety, but it may not be so for the gay person hiding in a military career; or for the young lesbian brought up in an Evangelical Christian family whose church tells her that she must change; or for the gay teen without social supports in a rural town and who is contemplating suicide as the only way out of his profound sense of isolation. We do not need to be heroic, but each of us needs to do the speaking out, teaching, research, or writing that will help these people and others. This is the obligation we have to our patients, to society, and to our mentors and forbears. To continue their work is our absolute duty and responsibility (Merlino, 2006).

REFERENCES

American Psychiatric Association (2005), Support of legal recognition of same sex civil marriage. Retrieved from http://www.psych.org/edu/other_res/lib_archives/archives/200502.pdf.

Drescher, J. (1998), *Psychoanalytic Therapy and the Gay Man.* Hillsdale, NJ: The Analytic Press.

Drescher, J. & Zucker, K.J., eds. (2006), *Ex-Gay Research: Analyzing the Spitzer Study and Its Relation to Science, Religion, Politics, and Culture.* Binghamton, NY: The Haworth Press.

Geltman, D. (2002), An interview with Arthur Kravitz, MD. *J. Gay & Lesbian Psychotherapy,* 6(4):97-105.

Melzer, E.J. (2005), Gay psychiatrist seeks APA presidency. *Washington Blade,* December 2. Retrieved from http://www.washblade.com/2005/12-2/news/national/gay-apa.cfm.

Merlino, J.P. (1997), Support groups for professional caregivers: A role for the contemporary psychoanalyst. *J. American Academy Psychoanalysis,* 25:111-122.

Merlino, J.P. (2001), An interview with Bertram H. Schaffner, M.D. *J. Gay & Lesbian Psychotherapy,* 5(1):85-99.

Merlino, J.P. (2006), Psychoanalysis and ethics: Relevant then, essential now. *J. American Academy Psychoanalysis & Dynamic Psychiatry,* 34(2):231-247.

Rosario, V.A. (2002), *Homosexuality and Science: A Guide to the Debates*. Santa Barbara, CA: ABC-CLIO.

Shidlo, A., Schroeder, M. & Drescher, J., eds. (2001), *Sexual Conversion Therapy: Ethical, Clinical and Research Perspectives*. Binghamton, NY: The Haworth Press.

Index

Page numbers followed by the letter "i" indicate illustrations; those followed by the letter "n" indicate notes.

doi:10.1300/6049_20

For Product Safety Concerns and Information please contact our EU representative GPSR@taylorandfrancis.com
Taylor & Francis Verlag GmbH, Kaufingerstraße 24, 80331 München, Germany

www.ingramcontent.com/pod-product-compliance
Lightning Source LLC
LaVergne TN
LVHW011114300926
849160LV00008B/378
* 9 7 8 1 5 6 0 2 3 7 3 9 6 *